GLOBAL POPULATION HEALTH

A PRIMER

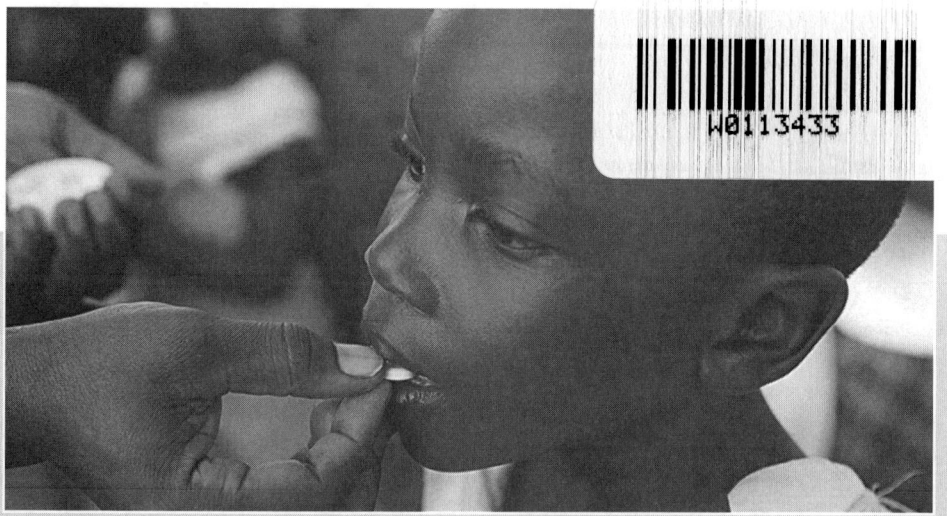

RICHARD SKOLNIK, MPA

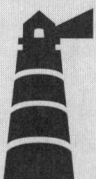

JONES & BARTLETT
LEARNING

World Headquarters
Jones & Bartlett Learning
25 Mall Road
Burlington, MA 01803
978-443-5000
info@jblearning.com
www.jblearning.com

Jones & Bartlett Learning books and products are available through most bookstores and online booksellers. To contact Jones & Bartlett Learning directly, call 800-832-0034, fax 978-443-8000, or visit our website, www .jblearning.com.

22526-6

Production Credits

Vice President, Product Management: Marisa R. Urbano
Vice President, Product Operations: Christine Emerton
Director, Product Management: Matthew Kane
Product Manager: Sophie Fleck Teague
Director, Content Management: Donna Gridley
Content Strategist: Sara Bempkins
Director, Project Management and Content Services: Karen Scott
Manager, Project Management: Jessica deMartin
Project Specialist: Roberta Sherman
Senior Digital Project Specialist: Angela Dooley

Senior Marketing Manager: Susanne Walker
Content Services Manager: Colleen Lamy
VP, Manufacturing and Inventory Control: Therese Connell
Composition: Exela Technologies
Project Management: Exela Technologies
Cover Design: Michael O'Donnell
Media Development Editor: Faith Brosnan
Rights & Permissions Manager: John Rusk
Rights Specialist: Rebecca Damon
Cover and Title Page Image: Courtesy of Mark Tuschman
Printing and Binding: McNaughton & Gunn

Library of Congress Cataloging-in-Publication Data
Names: Skolnik, Richard L. author.
Title: Global population health : a primer / Richard Skolnik.
Description: First edition. | Burlington, Massachusetts : Jones & Bartlett Learning, [2023] | Includes bibliographical references and index.
Identifiers: LCCN 2021025778 | ISBN 9781284175912 (paperback)
Subjects: MESH: Global Health | Population Health | Population Health Management | BISAC: MEDICAL / Public Health
Classification: LCC RA441 | NLM WA 530.1 | DDC 362.1--dc23 LC record available at https://lccn.loc.gov/2021025778

6048

Printed in the United States of America
26 25 24 23 22   10 9 8 7 6 5 4 3 2 1

Brief Contents

Contents

CHAPTER 3 **Health Systems and Universal Health Coverage** **30**

CHAPTER 4 **Environmental and Occupational Health and Intersectoral Approaches** **47**

CHAPTER 5 **Nutrition and the Health of Women, Children, Adolescents and Young Adults** **67**

Acknowledgments

A number of people were instrumental in the development of this book and I would like to thank and acknowledge them below.

Dick Riegelman, the Founding Dean and Professor of Epidemiology at The George Washington University Milken Institute School of Public Health, developed the idea of a series of public health primers. I appreciate Dick's inviting me to prepare a primer on global population health as part of the series. I am also grateful for Dick's continuous support of my efforts.

Hope Van Bronkhorst is a former student of mine at Yale and now a graduate student in public health at The George Washington University Milken Institute School of Public Health. Hope worked as my primary research assistant on this book. Among other things, she graciously and meticulously gathered data, prepared tables and figures, prepared shortened versions of case studies, and reviewed all that I wrote, at every stage of development and production.

Alison Zerbib is an undergraduate student at Yale University. Alison also worked as a research assistant on the book, focusing on the later stages of reviewing copyedits and page proofs.

Gary Bisbee is an outstanding copyeditor who reviewed all of the drafts of the book for me and helped to consolidate many different pieces into a harmonious whole.

Aviva Musius is a former student of mine at Yale who is a postdoctoral fellow at the Harvard T.C. Chan School of Public Health. Aviva was the co-author of the nutrition chapter of *Global Health 101, Fourth Edition*. Aviva helped me to adapt that chapter to this book.

Dr. Bente Moen, from the University of Bergen, kindly prepared the draft of the Occupational Health section of the book and worked with me to ensure its successful completion.

My thanks, as well, to all of the other people who helped me to write Global Health 101, without which this book would not have been possible.

I would also like to extend my thanks and appreciation to Sara Bempkins, Roberta Sherman, and Sophie Teague of Jones & Bartlett Learning. There cannot be a more supportive, talented, or gracious publishing team anywhere.

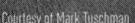

Introduction

Why Should We Care About Global Health?

The health of anyone, anywhere, is the health of everyone, everywhere and must, therefore, be a concern for all of us.

First, diseases do not respect boundaries, and globalization has increased the speed with which diseases can cross boundaries. The number of countries at risk of dengue or Chikungunya virus continues to increase. A novel coronavirus that erupted in China in 2019 began to wreak havoc throughout the world in only a few months.

Second, there is an ethical dimension to the health and well-being of other people. It is estimated that 5.2 million children under five years of age died in 2019, overwhelmingly from preventable causes.[1] In addition, many adults in poor countries die because they lack access to medicines that are typically available to people in rich countries. Is this fair? Are we prepared to accept such deaths without collectively taking steps to prevent them?

Third, health is closely linked with economic and social development in an increasingly interdependent world. Children who suffer from repeated illness and undernutrition may not reach their full biological or mental potential. Adults who suffer from HIV/AIDS, tuberculosis, malaria, and heart disease lose income while they are sick and out of work. Improving health enables individuals, their families, and their communities to fulfill more of their social and economic potential and to avoid poverty traps.

Finally, people's health and well-being have important implications for global security and freedom. For example, the cost of the 2014 Ebola outbreak in West Africa has been estimated at over $53 billion.[2] Early estimates of the economic consequences of COVID-19 suggested that the costs to the United States alone were already around $16 trillion dollars.[3]

The Aim of the Book

The aim of this book is to examine a range of the most critical global health topics in a brief, clear, and engaging manner. The book will provide the reader with an overview of the importance of global health, examine a number of the most important global health issues and their economic and social consequences, and discuss some of the steps that can be taken to address these concerns in cost-effective, fair, doable, and sustainable ways.

Key Guidance Questions

The book seeks to assist students in acquiring a basic understanding of global health. It focuses on readers gaining the knowledge needed to address five questions from an evidence-based and interdisciplinary perspective:

- *What is the problem?* This relates to what people get sick, disabled, and die from and how that varies by age, sex, income, and a number of other factors.
- *Who gets the problem?* This concerns which population groups are most affected.
- *Why do they get this problem?* What are the determinants of their morbidity and mortality?
- *Why should we care about this problem?* What is the relationship between these concerns and the opportunity of people, communities, and nations to realize their social and economic potential?
- *What can be done to address the problem?* What does the best evidence say can be done to address the problem at the lowest cost, as fast as possible, and in doable, sustainable, and fair ways?

The Perspective of the Book

The book is intended to be a brief introduction to global health. There are a number of important topics the book does not cover. Two of the most important are the history of global health and global health governance. Readers of this book are encouraged to pursue these and a number of other global health topics in other writings.

The book will take a *population health* perspective. Population health can be defined as:

> *the health outcomes of a group of individuals, including the distribution of such outcomes within the group.*[4]

The book will be global in perspective but will pay particular attention to low- and middle-income countries and low-income and marginalized people within them. The book will also focus considerable attention on universal health coverage; equity and health disparities; and the quality of health services. Another theme that runs through the book is the connection between health and social and economic development.

The book follows the point of view that health is a human right. The book is written with the presumption that governments have an obligation to try to ensure that all of their people have access to an affordable package of healthcare services and that all people should be protected from the costs of ill health. The book also follows from the principle that the aim of a health system is to *maximize the health of a population, at least cost, in the fairest possible ways.*

References

1. UNICEF, *Under-five mortality.* 2020. Retrieved from https://data.unicef.org/topic/child-survival/under-five-mortality

2. Huber C, Finelli L, Stevens W. The economic and social burden of the 2014 Ebola outbreak in West Africa. *J Infect Dis.* 2018;218(suppl 5):S698–S704. https://doi.org/10.1093/infdis/jiy213 Published 13 October 2018.

3. National Bureau of Economic Research (NBER). *David Cutler discusses the economic Cost of COVID-19.* November 16, 2020. Available at: https://www.nber.org/affiliated-scholars/researchspotlight/david-cutler-discusses-economic-cost-covid-19

4. Kindig D, Stoddart G. What is population health? *A J Public Health.* 2003;93(3):380–383.

CHAPTER 1

The Principles and Goals of Global Health

LEARNING OBJECTIVES

By the end of this chapter, the reader will be able to do the following:

- Define the terms health, public health, and global health
- Discuss some examples of public health efforts
- Discuss some examples of global health activities
- Describe some of the guiding principles of public health work, including a concern for equity, ethics, and ethical priority setting

VIGNETTES

Getachew is a 20-year-old Ethiopian with human immunodeficiency virus (HIV). He was recently placed on antiretroviral therapy for his infection. He is already gaining weight and feeling much stronger than before. Getachew is one of approximately 670,000 people in Ethiopia who are living with HIV.[1] He is also one of about 38 million people in the world who are HIV positive.[2] In Botswana, Lesotho, and Eswatini, more than 20% of all adults are HIV positive.[3]

Nirupama is a 50-year-old woman who lives in Chennai, India. Nirupama has diabetes. She is dependent on a regular supply of insulin. Although she is only 50, she has already suffered from some of the circulatory complications of diabetes. There is a common perception that diabetes is a disease that affects only people in high-income countries. This, however, is not the case.

Why Study Global Health?

Over the last 50 years, the world has made significant progress in improving human health.

As shown in **Table 1-1**, never before have so many people lived for so long, so few young children died each year, or so few women died each year of maternal causes. One reason to study global health is to gain a better understanding of the progress made so far in addressing global health problems.

Table 1-1 The Good News and the Unfinished Agenda in Global Health

Progress in Global Health	The Unfinished Agenda in Global Health
The number of polio cases globally has declined by approximately 99.99% since 1988 when the Global Polio Eradication Initiative (GPEI) was launched[1]	There were 5.2 million under five child deaths in 2019[6]
There were 38% fewer maternal deaths in 2017 than in 2000[2]	There were 295,000 maternal deaths in 2017[2]
There were 23% fewer new HIV infections in 2019 compared with 2010[3]	1.7 million people became infected with HIV in 2019[3]
The number of Guinea Worm cases has decreased over 99.9%, from 3.5 million in 1986 to 27 in 2020[4]	Approximately 1 billion people are infected with roundworm[7]
There were 60 million fewer tobacco users in 2018 than in 2000[5]	The prevalence of diabetes has doubled since 1980[8]

[1] Lickness JS, Gardner T, Diop OM, et al. Surveillance to Track Progress Toward Polio Eradication — Worldwide, 2018–2019. *Morbidity and Mortality Weekly Report (MMWR)*. 2020;69(20), 623-629. https://doi.org/10.15585/mmwr.mm6920a3
[2] World Health Organization, UNICEF, UNFPA, World Bank Group and the United Nations Population Division. *Trends in Maternal Mortality: 2000 to 2017*. Geneva: World Health Organization. 2019. https://data.unicef.org/resources/trends-maternal-mortality-2000-2017/
[3] UNAIDS. *Seizing the moment: tackling entrenched inequalities to end epidemics*. Geneva: UNAIDS. Retrieved December 23, 2020 from https://www.unaids.org/en/resources/documents/2020/global-aids-report
[4] The Carter Center. *Guinea Worm Case Totals*. 2020. Retrieved December 23, 2020 from https://www.cartercenter.org/health/guinea_worm/case-totals.html
[5] World Health Organization. WHO launches new report on global tobacco use trends. 2019. Retrieved December 23, 2020, from https://www.who.int/news/item/19-12-2019-who-launches-new-report-on-global-tobacco-use-trends
[6] UNICEF. *Levels and Trends in Child Mortality: Report 2020*. 2020. Retrieved June 23, 2021 from https://data.unicef.org/resources/levels-and-trends-in-child-mortality/
[7] Centers for Disease Control and Prevention. *Parasites – Ascariasis*. 2018. Retrieved July 22, 2018 from https://www.cdc.gov/parasites/ascariasis/index.html
[8] World Health Organization. *Global Report on Diabetes*. Geneva: World Health Organization. 2016. Retrieved July 22, 2018 from http://www.who.int/diabetes/global-report/en/

Another reason to study global health is to better understand the most important global health challenges that remain and how they might be addressed rapidly, effectively, efficiently, and fairly. Table 1-1 also describes some of the "unfinished agenda" of communicable diseases and neonatal, maternal, and nutritional causes of ill health. In addition, it speaks to the growing burden of noncommunicable diseases in low- and middle-income countries and the burden of injuries.

As the world becomes more globalized, the health of people everywhere must be of concern to all of us. This is particularly important because many diseases, such as tuberculosis (TB), HIV/AIDS, polio, dengue, and the coronaviruses, are not confined by political boundaries.

There are also disparities in the health of some groups compared with the health of others that raise important ethical concerns. Life expectancy in Japan, for example, is 84 years, but it is only 54 years in Sierra Leone.[4] In addition, there are a number of lifesaving technologies, such as the hepatitis B vaccine, that have been widely used in high-income countries for many years but are not yet disseminated as widely in low-income countries.

The important link between health and development is another reason to pay particular attention to global health. The poor health of mothers is linked to the poor health of babies and the failure of children to reach their full mental and physical potential. In addition, children's ill health can delay their entry into school and can affect their attendance, their academic performance, and their future economic prospects.

The intersectoral nature of many global health concerns and the need for different actors to work together to address them are additional reasons why we should be concerned with global health. Some problems, such as ensuring access to drugs to treat HIV/AIDS, require more financial resources than many individual countries can provide. Other global health issues require technical cooperation across countries. Global cooperation might be needed, for example, to establish standards for drug safety, set protocols for the treatment of certain health problems, develop an HIV vaccine, reduce anti-microbial resistance, or prepare for and act against pandemics.

Health, Public Health, and Global Health

Health

In 1946, the World Health Organization (WHO) established a definition of health that is still widely used, as it is in this text:

> Health is a state of complete physical, mental and social well-being and not merely the absence of disease or infirmity.[5]

Public Health

This book is mostly about public health and the health of populations. C.E.A. Winslow, considered to be the founder of modern public health in the United States, formulated a definition of public health in 1923 that is still commonly used today:

> The science and the art of preventing disease, prolonging life, and promoting physical health and mental health and efficiency through organized community efforts toward a sanitary environment; the control of community infections; the education of the individual in principles of personal hygiene; the organization of medical and nursing service for the early diagnosis and treatment of disease; and the development of the social machinery to ensure to every individual in the community a standard of living adequate for the maintenance of health.[6]

According to Winslow's definition, some examples of public health activities would include the development of a campaign to promote child immunization, an effort to get people to use seat belts when they drive, and actions to get people to eat healthier foods and to stop smoking tobacco. In addition, most levels of government also carry out certain public health functions, including the management of public health laboratories and clinics, the inspection of public eating establishments, and the maintenance of disease surveillance systems.

Many people confuse "public health" and "medicine," although they have quite different approaches.[7] To a large extent, the biggest difference between the medical approach and the public health approach is the focus in public health on the health of populations rather than on the health of individuals.[7]

Global Health

The U.S. National Academy of Medicine, earlier called the Institute of Medicine, defines global health as "health problems, issues, and concerns that transcend national boundaries and may best be addressed by cooperative actions."[8] Another group defined global health as "the application of the principles of public health to health problems and challenges that transcend national boundaries and to the complex array of global and local forces that affect them."[9]

Some examples of important global health concerns include the factors that contribute to women dying of pregnancy-related causes in so many countries; the exceptional amount of undernutrition among young children, especially in South Asia and sub-Saharan Africa; and the burden of different communicable and noncommunicable diseases worldwide and what can be done to control them. The impact of the environment on health globally and the effects of climate change, natural disasters, and conflicts are also important to global health. Other significant global health issues include how countries can organize and manage their health systems to enable the healthiest population possible given the resources available; the search for new technologies to address important global health problems; and how different actors can work together to solve health problems that no country or actor can solve on its own. Another global health matter of importance is the relationship between globalization and the health of different communities.

One Health

While this text focuses on global health, it will also deal in a number of sections with the concept of "**One Health**." The American Veterinary Medical Foundation defines One Health as follows:

> The integrative effort of multiple disciplines working locally, nationally, and globally to attain optimal health for people, animals, and the environment.[10]

Learners should note that the One Health approach is getting increasing attention among those working in global health. The 2019 coronavirus outbreak highlighted the importance of taking a One Health approach to a range of health issues.

Critical Global Health Concepts

Some of the most important global health concepts are:

- The **social determinants** and other determinants of health
- The key risk factors for different health conditions
- The global burden of disease
- The measurement of health status
- The demographic and epidemiologic transitions
- The organization and functions of health systems
- Links among health, education, development, poverty, and equity

Building on these concepts, those interested in global health also need to understand how key health issues, such as the following, affect different parts of the world:

- Environmental health
- Nutrition
- Reproductive health
- The health of children, adolescents, and young adults
- Communicable diseases
- Noncommunicable diseases and mental health disorders
- Injuries

Finally, it is important to understand global health issues that are generally addressed through cooperation. Some of these concern conflicts, natural disasters, and humanitarian emergencies.

Approaches to Global Health

There are a number of principles, frameworks, and questions that can be used to guide your study or work in global health, as noted below:

- It is valuable to think about health in a broad, multidisciplinary way.
- When working in global health, setting priorities will always be important.
- In low-income countries, where there is a heavy toll of death among young children, the health challenge, in many ways, is to "bury old people instead of young people, make the transition as fast as possible, and do it at the least cost."
- In high-income countries, in which people tend to live long lives, but often with many years of disability, the health challenge, in many ways, is to "help people live as long as possible and to spend those years in a healthy state."
- *How* countries spend money on health is often more important than *how much* they spend on health.

In addition, there are a number of questions that can guide your consideration of how to move from identifying global health issues to addressing them in sustainable, doable, fair, and cost-efficient ways:

- What is the problem?
- Who does the problem affect?
- What are the risk factors and determinants of the problem?

- Why should we care about this problem?
- What have we learned that can be done to address the problem in evidence-based, doable, sustainable, fair, and cost-efficient ways?

Equity and Health Disparities

Health inequity and health disparities are important public health concerns. Amartya Sen, a Nobel Laureate in Economics, has suggested that we should see **health equity** as multidimensional:

> It includes concerns about achievement of health and the capability to achieve good health, not just the distribution of health care. But it also includes the fairness of processes and thus must attach importance to non-discrimination in the delivery of health care.[11]

Sen has also suggested that health equity must be seen in the broader context of social justice issues, social structures within countries, and how countries choose to allocate their resources.[11]

A well-known British scholar of public health and the determinants of health, Margaret Whitehead, defines **health inequity** as "differences in health that are not only unnecessary and avoidable, but also unfair and unjust."[12]

Another important term relates to **inequality**. WHO defines health inequality as "differences in health status or in the distribution of health determinants between different population groups."[13]

Health disparities is another very commonly used term in public health and global health. The U.S. Centers for Disease Control and Prevention (CDC) defines health disparities as "a type of difference in health that is closely linked with social or economic disadvantage."[14] Although equity and equality are often used interchangeably when writing about health, in principle, equity concerns fairness, whereas equality largely refers to outcomes. It is essential to consider equity, inequality, and health disparities when discussing the different aspects of health care.

When taking an "equity, inequality, and health disparity lens" to global health concerns, it is also important to consider how such concerns vary according to the following factors:

- Social and economic status
- Health status and disability
- Ethnicity
- Gender
- Religion
- Location
- Occupation
- Social capital
- Sexual orientation

Additionally, it is important to keep in mind differences in key health issues both *across* and *within* countries.

To a large extent, the pattern of health disparities can be summarized relatively easily:

- Less-well-off people, with less social and political power, will generally have worse health, poorer health services, and less protection in the financing of health services than those who are better off.
- These less-well-off groups will generally include women; indigenous people; ethnic, religious, and other minority groups; the poor; those living in rural areas; those working in the informal sector of the economy; those with limited education; and those who have relatively lower levels of social capital. Generally, disabled people; people with mental illness; and lesbian, gay, bisexual, and transgender people will also face discrimination that leads to inequities, inequalities, and disparities in health.

Health and Human Rights

There is an extremely important connection between health and human rights, and health priorities must be set in ethical ways. Painful ethical dilemmas arise in the pursuit of global health, whether in planning a healthcare provision, implementing public health measures, or conducting health research. It is important to address these issues, both for their own sake and because there is a strong complementarity between good ethical and human rights practices and good health outcomes.[15]

International conventions and treaties recognize access to health services and health information as human rights. Yet, in many countries, there are remarkable gaps in access to health services. The poor and the disenfranchised suffer from these gaps the most.

The failure to respect human rights is often associated with harm to human health. This has frequently been the case, for example, with diseases that are highly stigmatized, such as leprosy, TB, and HIV/AIDS. If leprosy patients are not provided with the best care because some health workers are afraid to work with them, the leprosy patients cannot stop the progression of their disease. If TB patients are shunned by health workers, they may die, usually after infecting many other people.

Efforts to maintain public health while dealing with new and emerging diseases, such as a novel coronavirus, raise another array of ethical and human rights issues. When we face a potential health threat, for example, what are the rights of individuals compared with the rights of society to protect its members from illness? Is it acceptable to quarantine a city? Is it permissible to ban travel? Can a government mandate the use of face masks? These are real issues with which policymakers and health practitioners must wrestle, as seen vividly during the COVID-19 pandemic.

Another set of ethical issues is associated with research on human subjects. Health research involving people is generally considered ethically challenging because, in contrast to clinical care, research participants are put at risk for the sake of other people's health. An important part of the research that takes place in the pursuit of global health must also deal with further ethical concerns that arise when research is conducted with poor people who do not have access to satisfactory levels of health care outside of a research study.

Finally, it is important to ensure that health investments are made in fair ways. Even in high-income countries, the resources available for health care are limited. How can choices about who should live and who should die be fair and perceived as legitimate? In low- and middle-income countries, where there are fewer resources and greater needs, difficult decisions must constantly be made about which populations and diseases should get priority. Recent developments in ethical theory can help illuminate such difficult choices.

The Organization of Data in This Text

This text presents most data in terms of country income level. The World Bank classifies countries into four income groups based on estimates of their gross national income (GNI) per capita. For the World Bank's 2021 fiscal year, country income groups are defined as noted below. You can also see below some countries that fall in those income categories:

- Low-income economies: GNI per capita of $1,035 or less—Afghanistan, Ethiopia, Haiti
- Lower middle-income economies: GNI per capita between $1,036 and $4,035—Bangladesh, Bolivia, India
- Upper middle-income economies: GNI per capita between $4,046 and $12,535—Argentina, Costa Rica, Turkey
- High-income economies: GNI per capita of $12,536 or more—Belgium, Canada, Portugal[16]

The text presents some data by World Bank Region or region of WHO.

This text contains considerable information on the burden of disease and attributable risk factors. This information is drawn largely from the *Global Burden of Diseases, Injuries, and Risk Factors Study, 2019* (*GBD 2019*), which was prepared by the Institute of Health Metrics and Evaluation (IHME). Findings of the study have been published in a series of articles in *The Lancet*.[17] Much of the data from that study are also presented on the extensive and interactive burden of disease website of the IHME.[18] This text will refer to the study and all of its related parts as *The Global Burden of Disease Study 2019*, *GBD 2019*, or *GBD*.

The burden of disease data from the IHME study is complemented as needed by data published by other organizations, such as UNICEF, WHO, and the World Bank, and from data published in *Disease Control Priorities in Developing Countries, Second Edition*[19] and *Third Edition*.[20]

The Sustainable Development Goals

The 17 Sustainable Development Goals (SDGs) were formulated by the global community in 2015 as part of the 2030 Agenda for Sustainable Development.[21] **Figure 1-1** portrays the 17 SDGs.

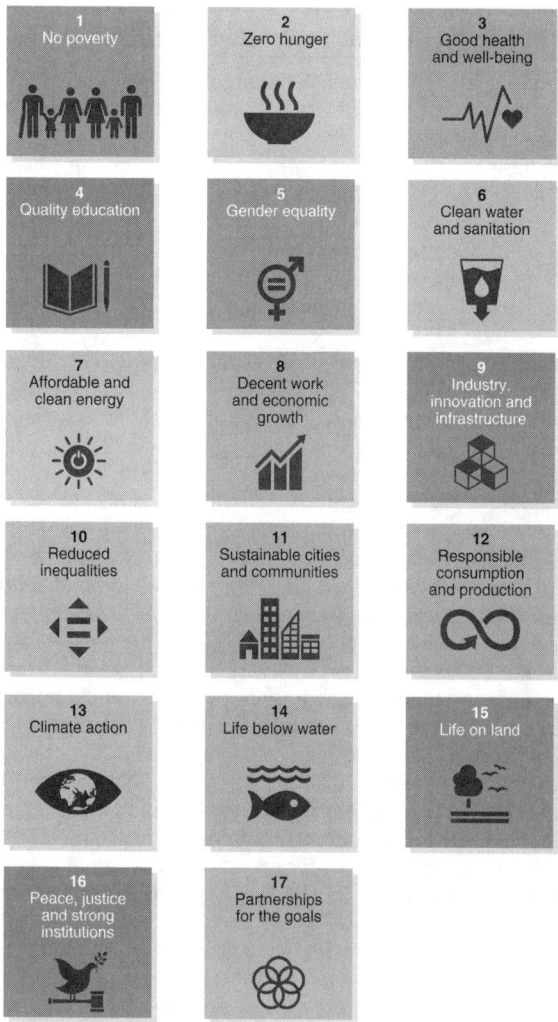

Figure 1-1 Sustainable Development Goals

Some of the SDGs have a very direct link with health, such as Goal 3—"ensure healthy life and promote well-being for all at all ages." Others have a less direct but still very important link with the achievement of good health: Goal 1: No poverty; Goal 2: Zero Hunger; Goal 4: Quality Education; Goal 6: Clean water and sanitation. In addition to the above goals, it is easy to see how all of the goals have an important, even if indirect, relationship with the achievement of good health and well-being.

Most of the goals also have an associated set of specific targets that are to be achieved by 2020 or 2030. The targets for Goal 3—"to ensure healthy lives and promote well-being for all at all ages"—are shown in **Table 1-2**.

Table 1-2 Targets for Sustainable Development in Achieving Goal 3

- By 2030, end the epidemics of AIDS, tuberculosis, malaria, and neglected tropical diseases; and combat hepatitis, waterborne diseases, and other communicable diseases.
- By 2030, reduce by one-third premature mortality from noncommunicable diseases through prevention and treatment and promote mental health and well-being.
- Strengthen the prevention and treatment of substance abuse, including narcotic drug abuse and harmful use of alcohol.
- By 2020, halve the number of global deaths and injuries from road traffic accidents.
- By 2030, ensure universal access to sexual and reproductive healthcare services, including for family planning, information and education, and the integration of reproductive health into national strategies and programs.
- Achieve universal health coverage, including financial risk protection; access to quality essential healthcare services; and access to safe, effective, quality, and affordable essential medicines and vaccines for all.
- By 2030, substantially reduce the number of deaths and illnesses from hazardous chemicals and air, water, and soil pollution and contamination.
- Strengthen the implementation of the World Health Organization Framework Convention on Tobacco Control in all countries, as appropriate.
- Support the research and development of vaccines and medicines for the communicable and noncommunicable diseases that primarily affect developing countries, and provide access to affordable essential medicines and vaccines in accordance with the Doha Declaration on the TRIPS Agreement and Public Health, which affirms the right of developing countries to use the full provisions in the Agreement on Trade-Related Aspects of Intellectual Property Rights regarding flexibilities to protect public health, and in particular, provide access to medicines for all.
- Substantially increase health financing and the recruitment, development, training, and retention of the health workforce in developing countries, especially in least developed countries and small island developing states.
- Strengthen the capacity of all countries, in particular developing countries, for early warning, risk reduction, and management of national and global health risks.

United Nations Sustainable Development Goals Knowledge Platform. nd *Sustainable Development Goals.* © United Nations. Reprinted with the permission of the United Nations.

Central Messages of This Text

This chapter ends by highlighting some of the central messages of the text as a whole.

- The health of anyone, anywhere, is the health of everyone, everywhere.
- People's health is shaped by a range of determinants, including political, economic, and social determinants, as well as exposure to risk factors.

- An important part of health status is determined by an individual's and family's knowledge of health and hygiene.
- Historical, political, and social forces have helped to shape health issues and the development of health systems in all countries.
- Most countries regard health as a human right and seek to achieve a system of universal health coverage.
- There are strong links among health, human development, labor productivity, and economic development.
- There has been enormous progress in improving health status over the last 50 years.
- Some of this progress has come about as a result of overall economic development and improvements in income. However, much of it is due to improvements in public hygiene, better water supply and sanitation, and better education. Increased nutritional status has also had a large impact on improvements in health status. Technical progress in some areas, such as the development and dissemination of vaccines against childhood diseases and antibiotics, has also improved human health.
- There are proven packages of investments that can address a range of issues related to neonatal, maternal, and child health, and communicable diseases. However, they have not yet been taken to sufficient scale in many low- and middle-income countries.
- There is an increasing amount of evidence about measures that can be taken, on a large scale, to reduce the risk of and address noncommunicable diseases in cost-effective ways. However, many low- and middle-income countries are only now beginning to take steps to reduce the burden of noncommunicable diseases. Many high-income countries have also failed to address these issues effectively at scale.
- The progress in improving health status has been very uneven. Hundreds of millions of people, especially poor people in low- and middle-income countries, continue to get sick, be disabled by, or die from preventable diseases.
- There are enormous disparities in health status and access to health services both within and across countries. These vary by income, location, ethnicity, religion, occupation, sex, and sexual orientation, among other factors.
- There are exceptional gaps in the quality of health services everywhere, but especially in low- and middle-income countries.
- Countries do not need to be high-income to enjoy good health status, as reflected by China, Costa Rica, Cuba, Kerala state in India, and Sri Lanka, among others.
- When considering health policy, one must always seek the most value for the money available and ask: "If we only had $100 to spend, how should we spend it to achieve the maximum health for our people, at least cost, and in doable, sustainable, and fair ways?"
- The burden of disease globally is predominantly noncommunicable and evolving in light of economic and social changes, aging populations, and scientific and technical progress, among other things.
- Some global health issues can only be solved through the cooperation of various actors in global health. This could include, for example, the eradication of polio.

- Taking account of these points, we could say, in many respects, that low-income countries should focus on "burying old people, instead of young people, making the transition as fast as possible, and doing so at least cost and in fair ways."
- Taking account of these points, we could also say, in many respects, that the health goals for all countries are to "enable the maximum health for their people, in fairly distributed ways, at least cost."

Discussion Questions

1. Why should global health issues be important to everyone?
2. What are some of the most important factors related to health disparities?
3. What are some of the most important ethical concerns that relate to global health?
4. What factors led some countries to achieve rapid improvements in population health, even as they remained low-income countries?
5. How might the health goals of a high-income country differ from those of a low-income country and why?

References

1. UNAIDS. *Country|Ethiopia.* 2019. Retrieved from https://www.unaids.org/en/regionscountries/countries/ethiopia
2. UNAIDS. *Global HIV & AIDS statistics – 2019 fact sheet.* nd. Retrieved from https://www.unaids.org/en/resources/fact-sheet
3. Statista. Ranking of countries with the highest prevalence of HIV in 2000 and 2019. 2020. Retrieved from https://www.statista.com/statistics/270209/countries-with-the-highest-global-hiv-prevalence/
4. World Bank|Data. *Life expectancy at birth, total, (years).* nd. Retrieved from: https://data.worldbank.org/indicator/SP.DYN.LE00.IN
5. World Health Organization. *Preamble to the Constitution of the World Health Organization 1946, as adopted by the International Health Conference, New York, 19 June 22–July 1946.* 1946. Retrieved from http://apps.who.int/gb/bd/PDF/bd47/EN/constitution-en.pdf
6. Merson MH, Black RE, Mills A. *International public health: diseases, programs, systems, and policies* (p. xvii). Gaithersburg, MD: Aspen Publishers; 2001.
7. Harvard School of Public Health. *Distinctions between medicine and public health.* nd. Retrieved from http://www.hsph.harvard.edu/about/public-health-medicine/
8. Institute of Medicine. *America's vital interest in global health: Protecting our people, enhancing our economy, and advancing our international interests.* Washington, DC: National Academy Press; 1998.
9. Merson MH, Black RE, Mills A. *International public health: diseases, programs, systems, and policies* (p. xix). Gaithersburg, MD: Aspen Publishers; 2001.
10. American Veterinary Medical Foundation (AVMA). *One Health—It's all connected.* nd. Retrieved from https://www.avma.org/resources-tools/one-health. Retrieved June 29, 2021.
11. Sen A. Why health equity? *Health Economics.* 2002;11(8):665–666.
12. Whitehead M. The concepts and principles of equity and health. *International Journal of Health Services.* 1991;22(3):217–228.
13. World Health Organization. *Health inequities and their causes. 22 Feb 2018. Health impact assessment. Glossary of terms used.* nd. Retrieved June 23, 2021 from https://www.who.int/news-room/facts-in-pictures/detail/health-inequities-and-their-causes

14. Centers for Disease Control and Prevention. *Defining and measuring disparities, inequities, and inequalities in the Health People Initiative*. nd. Retrieved from http://www.cdc.gov/social determinants/Definitions.html

15. Mann, J, Gostin L, Gruskin S, Brennan T, Lazzarini Z, Fineberg H. Health and human rights. *Health and Human Rights*. 1994:1(1), 6–23.

16. The World Bank. *Data. World Bank Country and Lending Groups*. nd. Available at: https://datahelpdesk.worldbank.org/knowledgebase/articles/906519-world-bank-country-and-lending-groups

17. The Lancet. *Global Burden of Disease*. 2020. Available at: https://www.thelancet.com/gbd#2019GBDIssue. https://www.thelancet.com/journals/lancet/issue/vol396no10258/PIIS0140-6736(20)X0042-0

18. Institute of Health Metrics and Evaluation (IHME). GBD Compare: Viz Hub. nd. Retrieved from https://vizhub.healthdata.org/gbd-compare/

19. Jamison, DEA. (Ed.). *Disease control priorities in developing countries* (2nd ed.). New York, NY: Oxford University Press and the World Bank; 2006.

20. Jamison DT, Nugent R, Gelband H, Horton S, Jha P, Laxminarayan R. (Eds.). *Disease control priorities: improving health and reducing poverty* (3rd ed., Vol. 9). Washington, DC: The World Bank; 2018.

21. United Nations. Sustainable Development Goals. nd. Retrieved from https://www.un.org/sustainabledevelopment/

CHAPTER 2

Health Determinants, Measurements, and the Global Burden of Disease

LEARNING OBJECTIVES

By the end of this chapter, the reader will be able to do the following:

- Describe the determinants of health
- Define the most important health indicators and key terms related to measuring health status and the burden of disease
- Discuss the status of health globally and how it varies by country income group, sex, and age group
- Discuss the burden of disease and how it varies by country income group, age, and sex
- Review major demographic patterns and the effect they have on the burden of disease

VIGNETTES

Maria is a poor Quechua woman who lives in the highlands of Peru. In Peru, poor people tend to live in the mountains, be indigenous, be less educated, and have worse health status than others. To understand and address differences in health status among different groups, how do we measure health status—by age, gender, socioeconomic status, level of education, ethnicity, location?

Abdul is a 4-year-old boy in northern India. For every 1,000 children born in South Asia in 2019, approximately 40 will die before their 5th birthday. The rate of child death is even higher in sub-Saharan Africa, at 76 per 1,000 live births.[1] What are the leading causes of death for young children like Abdul? What are the most important risk factors for those causes?

The Importance of Measuring Health Status

If we want to understand the most important global health issues and what can be done to address them, we must understand what factors have the most influence on health status, how health status is measured, and what people get sick, disabled, and die from.

The Determinants and Social Determinants of Health

People's health status depends on a large number of factors, many of which are interconnected, and most of which go considerably beyond access to health services.

The **determinants of health** can be defined as the "the range of personal, social, economic, and environmental factors that influence health status."[2] WHO defines the social determinants of health as the "conditions in which people are born, grow, live, work and age."[3]

Figure 2-1 shows one way of depicting the determinants of health. As we think about the determinants of health, we should be aware that increasing attention is being paid to the social determinants of health. We should also note the importance of health to child development, including the ways in which families nourish and care for infants and young children, beginning at conception. Being born premature or of low birth weight can have important negative consequences on health over

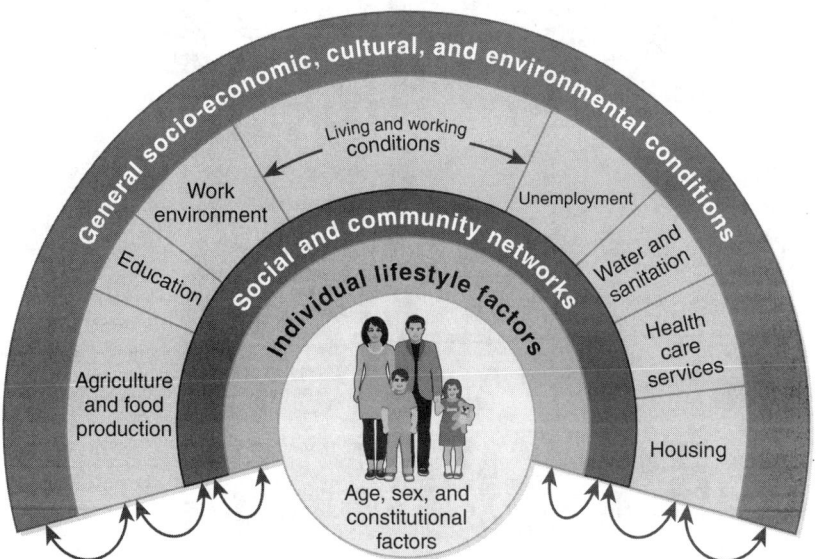

Figure 2-1 The Determinants of Health

Reproduced from Dahlgren G., & Whitehead M. (1991). *Policies and strategies to promote social equity in health*. Stockholm, Sweden: Institute for Futures Studies. Retrieved from http://www.iffs.se/media/1326/20080109110739filmZ8UVQv2wQFShMRF6cuT.pdf

the life course. There is a strong correlation between the nutritional status of infants and young children and the extent to which they meet their biological and intellectual potential, enroll in school, or stay in school. In addition, poor nutritional status in infancy and early childhood may be linked to a number of noncommunicable diseases later in life, including diabetes and heart disease.[4] Moreover, there is considerable evidence that a range of stressors, including poverty, abuse, and discrimination, have a powerful impact on the health of children that may continue through adulthood. [5]

Finally, as we think about the determinants, including the social determinants of health, it is important to consider how different factors influence health in indirect and direct ways. One framework for such consideration is shown in **Figure 2-2**.

Key Health Indicators

It is critical that we use data and evidence to understand and address key global health issues.

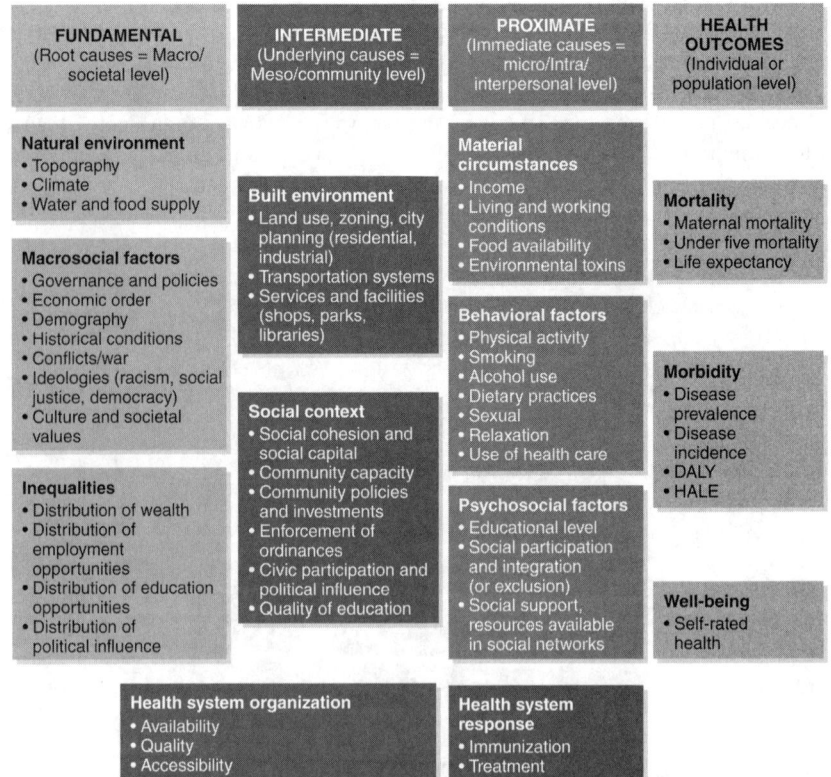

Figure 2-2 Selected Examples of Root, Underlying, and Immediate Determinants of Health

Modified with permission from Bouwman L., Wentink C., & Ormond M. (2017, April 6). Global Health, W3 Tutorial 3: Determinants [Powerpoint Slides]. Based on Northridge.

There are many important uses of data on health status.[6] We need data, for example, to know what health conditions cause people to be sick, disabled, or die. We need data to carry out disease surveillance. Other forms of data also help us to understand the burden of different health conditions and their relative importance to different societies.

It is also important that we use a consistent set of indicators to measure health status. The indicators that are used most commonly by those who work in global health are defined in **Table 2-1**.

Examining these key indicators by country income group or region highlights a number of points, including:

- There is a very strong correlation between country income group and health status. Generally, the lower the income group, the lower the health status; the higher the income group, the higher the health status.
- Sub-Saharan Africa has the worst health indicators of all World Bank regions, and South Asia has the second worst health indicators.

Part of the relatively low health status of sub-Saharan Africa and South Asia is related to the fact that these are the two regions with the lowest per capita income. However, their relatively low health status also has to do with government policies and programs, the lack of safe water and sanitation, low levels of education, and a number of other factors.

Even so, it is important to understand that country income level does not have to determine a country's health status. Rather, resource-poor countries that make wise policy choices in fair ways *can* enable better health for their people than their income level might suggest. This has certainly been the case for a number of countries whose development history is well known, such as China, Cuba, and Sri Lanka.

Among the most commonly used indicators of health status is **life expectancy at birth**. Generally, the higher the life expectancy at birth, the better the

---

Table 2-1 Key Health Status Indicators

Infant mortality rate: The number of deaths of infants under age 1 per 1,000 live births in a given year

Life expectancy at birth: The average number of years a newborn baby could expect to live if current mortality trends were to continue for the rest of the newborn's life

Maternal mortality ratio: The number of women who die as a result of pregnancy and childbirth complications per 100,000 live births in a given year

Neonatal mortality rate: The number of deaths of infants under 28 days of age in a given year per 1,000 live births in that year

Under five mortality rate (child mortality rate): The probability that a newborn baby will die before reaching age 5, expressed as a number per 1,000 live births

Modified from Soubbotina TP (2004). Glossary. In *Beyond economic growth: An introduction to sustainable development*. Washington, DC: The World Bank. Retrieved from http://documents.worldbank.org/curated/en/454041468780615049/Beyond -economic-growth-an-introduction-to-sustainable-development

health status of a country. Life expectancy at birth by country income group in 2019 was as follows: low-income, 64 years; lower middle-income, 69 years; upper middle-income, 76 years; and high-income, 81 years.[7]

The **maternal mortality ratio** is a measure of the risk of death that is associated with pregnancy and childbirth. Very few women die in childbirth in rich countries; for example, the maternal mortality ratio in Sweden in 2017 was 4 per 100,000 live births. On the other hand, in very poor countries, the ratios can be over 700 per 100,000 live births.[8]

Another important indicator is the **infant mortality rate**. This rate varies largely with the income status of a country. Many of the poorest countries in Africa have infant mortality rates greater than 60 deaths per 1,000 live births. However, in Sweden only about two infants die for every 1,000 live births.[9]

The infant mortality rate is a powerful indicator. However, most children younger than one year of age who die do so in the first month of life. Thus, the **neonatal mortality rate** is also an important health status indicator. The neonatal mortality rate across country income groups in 2019 was 27 deaths per 1,000 live births in low-income, 24 in lower middle-income, 7 in upper middle-income; and 3 in high-income.[10]

The under-5 child mortality rate is also called the **child mortality rate**. In the highest-income countries, the rate is generally about 3 to 5 per 1,000 live births. In some of the poorest countries, however, the rate is over 80 and in a few countries, it is over 100.[1]

There are a few other concepts and definitions that are important to understand as we think about measuring health status. The first is **morbidity**, which means sickness or any departure, subjective or objective, from a psychological or physiological state of well-being. Second is **mortality**, which refers to death. A **death rate** is the number of deaths per 1,000 population in a given year.[11] The third is **disability**, referring to the "temporary or long-term reduction in a person's capacity to function."[11]

There will also be considerable discussion in most readings on global health of the **prevalence** of health conditions. This refers to the number of people suffering from a certain health condition over a specific time period.[12]

The **incidence rate** measures how many people get a disease, for a specified number of people at risk, and for a given period of time.[12] In India, for example, the incidence rate for tuberculosis (TB) in 2019 was 193 per 100,000 people.[13] This means that for every 100,000 people in India, 193 got active TB disease in 2019.

Finally, one needs to be familiar with how diseases get classified. Some are **communicable diseases**, which are also called infectious diseases. These are illnesses that are caused by a particular infectious agent and that spread directly or indirectly from people to people, animals to people, or people to animals.[11] Examples of communicable diseases include influenza, measles, and HIV. **Noncommunicable diseases** are illnesses that are not spread by any infectious agent, such as hypertension, coronary heart disease, and diabetes, even though they might have an infectious cause, as cervical cancer has. **Injuries** include, among other things, road traffic injuries, falls, drownings, poisonings, and violence.[14]

Measuring the Burden of Disease

Those who work on global health have attempted for a number of years to construct a single indicator that could be used to compare how far different countries are from a state of good health. This kind of index would measure what is generally referred to as the **burden of disease**.

The composite indicator of health status that is most commonly used in global health work is called the **disability-adjusted life year**, or **DALY**. In the simplest terms, a DALY is "the sum of years lost due to premature death (YLLs) and years lived with disability (YLDs). DALYs are also defined as years of healthy life lost."[15]

The calculation of years lost to premature death is based on the difference between the age at which one dies and one's life expectancy at that age. To make this calculation, those involved in the key studies on the global burden of disease have constructed a reference standard **life table** that takes account of the highest life expectancy at birth globally. For the 2016 study, for example, this was set at 86.6 years.[16] The standard life table is used to calculate premature death for all countries in the study. The value for years lived with disability is calculated by multiplying the number of years lived with disability by a weight assigned to that disability.[17]

A society that has more premature death, illness, and disability has more DALYs per person in the population than a society that is healthier and has less premature death, illness, and disability. One of the goals of health policy is to avert these DALYs in the most cost-efficient and fair manner possible. An important point to remember when considering DALYs, compared with measuring deaths, is that DALYs take account of periods in which people are living with disability. By doing this, DALYs give a better estimate of the true health of a population than one would get measuring deaths alone.

For example, contrary to popular belief, mental health problems *are* associated with an important number of deaths. However, they also cause an enormous amount of disability. Several parasitic infections, such as schistosomiasis, cause very few deaths but large amounts of illness and disability. If we measured the health of a population with a significant burden of schistosomiasis and mental illness only by measuring deaths, we would miss a major component of morbidity and disability and would seriously overestimate the health of that population.

Burden of Disease Data

It is important to get a clear picture of the leading causes of death and disability in the world and how they vary by age, sex, ethnicity, and socioeconomic status, both within and across countries. Additionally, it is essential to understand how these causes have varied over time and how they might change in the future. Much of the data that follow on the burden of disease and risk factors is based on the findings of the Global Burden of Disease

Study 2019, published in *The Lancet* in 2020.[18] The Institute of Health Metrics and Evaluation (IHME) coordinated that study. This chapter also heavily uses data from interactive data visualizations that the IHME has posted on its website.[14] The reader should note that while some data refer to "deaths" and some data refer to "DALYs," references to the "burden of disease" refer to DALYs.

Earlier burden of disease studies categorized causes of deaths and DALYs by three groups, a construct that remains useful and is employed in this book:

- Group I—Communicable, maternal and perinatal conditions (meaning in the first week after birth), and nutritional disorders
- Group II—Noncommunicable diseases
- Group III—Injuries, including, among other things, road traffic accidents, falls, self-inflicted injuries, and violence

Overview of Patterns and Trends in the Burden of Disease

Some of the main findings of the burden of disease studies are summarized here. These findings do not take account of COVID-19.[18]

- People in much of the world are living longer than before, with women living 5 years longer than men.
- Globally, mortality rates have decreased for all age groups, with very substantial decreases for children under five years of age.
- Nonetheless, there are substantial differences in the rate of mortality decrease across countries.
- The years of life lost due to premature death are increasing for diabetes, some cancers, and, in some places, for drug use disorders, conflict, and terrorism.
- In the last 4 decades, there have been significant declines in communicable, maternal, neonatal, and nutritional causes of death.
- The burden of disease has shifted increasingly toward noncommunicable diseases and is predominantly noncommunicable in all World Bank regions and for all World Bank country income groups, except sub-Saharan Africa and low-income countries.
- This shift has been fueled by, among other things, a reduction in communicable diseases and the aging of populations.
- The five leading causes of deaths globally in 2019 were ischemic heart disease; stroke; chronic obstructive pulmonary disease; lower respiratory infections; and tracheal, bronchus, and lung cancer.
- As life expectancies increase, death rates decline, and populations age, there is an increase in the number of years people live with disability; this has increased as a share of the total burden of disease.
- Globally, low back pain, depressive disorders, headache disorders, age-related hearing loss, and iron-deficiency anemia were the five leading causes of years lived with disability in 2019.

- Globally, the top five risk factors for the burden of disease in 2019 were high blood pressure, particulate matter, smoking, high fasting plasma glucose, and low birth weight and short gestation.
- There are a number of countries in which life expectancy is greater than one might predict on the basis of social and economic development. These countries could provide useful lessons for other countries that have not made such progress in health.

The Leading Causes of Deaths and DALYs

The comments that follow provide some additional information about how the burden of deaths varies among under-5 children by country income group. This section also examines how the burden of both deaths and DALYs vary for people 15–49 years old and between females and males by country income group. These can serve as examples of how the burden of deaths and DALYs vary by age, sex, and country income group.

Table 2-2 shows the five leading causes of death for children aged 0 to 5 years by country income group.

Table 2-2 Five Leading Causes of Death Under Five Years of Age by World Bank Country Income Group, 2019

Rank	Cause			
	Low-Income	Lower Middle-Income	Upper Middle-Income	High-Income
1	Neonatal disorders	Neonatal disorders	Neonatal disorders	Neonatal disorders
2	Lower respiratory infections	Lower respiratory infections	Congenital defects	Congenital defects
3	Malaria	Diarrheal diseases	Lower respiratory infections	SIDS
4	Diarrheal diseases	Congenital defects	Diarrheal diseases	Foreign body
5	Congenital defects	Malaria	Foreign body	Lower respiratory infections

Data from Institute of Health Metrics and Evaluation (IHME). nd GBD Compare: Viz Hub. Retrieved from https://vizhub.healthdata.org/gbd-compare/

Table 2-3 examines the five leading causes of deaths and DALYs for the age group 15 to 49 by World Bank country income group.

Table 2-3 Five Leading Causes of Deaths and DALYs, 15–49, Both Sexes, by World Bank Country Income Group, 2019

Low-Income Countries

Cause

Rank	Deaths	DALYs
1	HIV/AIDS	HIV/AIDS
2	Tuberculosis	Tuberculosis
3	Maternal disorders	Road injuries
4	Road injuries	Maternal disorders
5	Diarrheal diseases	Depressive disorders

Lower Middle-Income Countries

Cause

Rank	Deaths	DALYs
1	Ischemic heart disease	Road injuries
2	Road injuries	Ischemic heart disease
3	Tuberculosis	Tuberculosis
4	HIV/AIDS	Headache disorders
5	Cirrhosis	HIV/AIDS

Upper Middle-Income Countries

Cause

Rank	Deaths	DALYs
1	Road injuries	Road injuries
2	HIV/AIDS	Interpersonal violence
3	Ischemic heart disease	Headache disorders
4	Interpersonal violence	HIV/AIDS
5	Stroke	Low back pain

High-Income Countries		
Cause		
Rank	**Deaths**	**DALYs**
1	Self-harm	Low back pain
2	Road injuries	Drug use disorders
3	Drug use disorders	Headache disorders
4	Ischemic heart disease	Depressive disorders
5	Cirrhosis	Road injuries

Data from Institute of Health Metrics and Evaluation (IHME). nd GBD Compare: Viz Hub. Retrieved from https://vizhub.healthdata.org/gbd-compare/

Causes of Deaths and DALYs by Sex

Table 2-4 examines DALYs by sex and by country income group in 2019.

Table 2-4 Five Leading Causes of DALYs, Males and Females, All Ages, by World Bank Country Income Group, 2019

Low-Income Countries		
Cause		
Rank	**Male**	**Female**
1	Neonatal disorders	Neonatal disorders
2	Diarrheal diseases	Lower respiratory infections
3	Lower respiratory infections	Malaria
4	Malaria	Diarrheal diseases
5	Tuberculosis	HIV/AIDS
Lower Middle-Income Countries		
Cause		
Rank	**Male**	**Female**
1	Neonatal disorders	Neonatal disorders
2	Ischemic heart disease	Ischemic heart disease
3	Lower respiratory infections	Diarrheal diseases
4	Stroke	Lower respiratory infections
5	Diarrheal diseases	Stroke

(continues)

Table 2-4 Five Leading Causes of DALYs, Males and Females, All Ages, by World Bank Country Income Group, 2019 *(continued)*

Upper Middle-Income Countries

Cause

Rank	Male	Female
1	Ischemic heart disease	Stroke
2	Stroke	Ischemic heart disease
3	Road injuries	Low back pain
4	Tracheal, bronchus, and lung cancer	Diabetes
5	COPD	COPD

High-Income Countries

Cause

Rank	Male	Female
1	Ischemic heart disease	Ischemic heart disease
2	Tracheal, bronchus, and lung cancer	Low back pain
3	Low back pain	Stroke
4	Stroke	Diabetes
5	Diabetes	Alzheimer's disease and other dementias

Data from Institute of Health Metrics and Evaluation (IHME). nd GBD Compare: Viz Hub. Retrieved from https://vizhub.healthdata.org/gbd-compare/

The Burden of Deaths and Disease Within Countries

As you consider causes of death and the burden of disease globally and by country income group, region, age, and sex, it is also important to consider how deaths and DALYs vary within countries by gender, ethnicity, and socioeconomic status, among other things. Generally speaking, the following statements are true:

- Rural populations will be less healthy than urban populations.
- Disadvantaged ethnic minorities will be less healthy than majority populations.
- Females will suffer a number of conditions that relate to their relatively disadvantaged social positions.
- Lower-income people will be less healthy than better-off people.
- Uneducated people will be less healthy than better-educated people.

In addition, people of lower socioeconomic status will have higher rates of communicable diseases, illness, and death related to maternal causes and malnutrition than people of higher socioeconomic status. People of lower socioeconomic status will also suffer from a larger burden of disease related to smoking, alcohol, and poor diet than would be the case for better-off people. These points are fundamental to understanding global health.

Risk Factors

A **risk factor** is "an aspect or personal behavior or lifestyle, an environmental exposure, or an inborn or inherited characteristic, that, on the basis of epidemiologic evidence, is known to be associated with health-related condition(s) considered important to prevent."[11] Risks that relate to health can also be thought of as "a probability of an adverse outcome, or a factor that raises this probability."[11]

It is very important to understand the risk factors to which health problems relate. **Table 2-5** shows the relative importance of different risk factors for deaths for different country income groups. **Table 2-6** does the same for DALYs. The burden of disease studies generally refer to these risks in three categories: behavioral, environmental and occupational, and metabolic.[18]

Table 2-5 Five Leading Risk Factors for Deaths, Globally, All Ages and Both Sexes, by World Bank Country Income Group, 2019

Risk Factor				
Rank	Low-Income	Lower Middle-Income	Upper-Middle Income	High-Income
1	Particulate matter	High blood pressure	High blood pressure	High blood pressure
2	High blood pressure	Particulate matter	Smoking	Smoking
3	Low birth weight and short gestation	High fasting plasma glucose	Particulate matter	High fasting plasma glucose
4	Child growth failure	Smoking	High fasting plasma glucose	High body-mass index
5	Unsafe water	High body-mass index	High body-mass index	High LDL

Data from Institute of Health Metrics and Evaluation (IHME). nd GBD Compare: Viz Hub. Retrieved from https://vizhub.healthdata.org/gbd-compare/

Table 2-6 Five Leading Risk Factors for DALYs, Globally, All Ages and Both Sexes, by World Bank Country Income Group, 2019

Risk Factor				
Rank	Low-Income	Lower Middle-Income	Upper-Middle Income	High-Income
1	Low birth weight and short gestation	Particulate matter	High blood pressure	Smoking
2	Child growth failure	Low birth weight and short gestation	Smoking	High body-mass index
3	Particulate matter	High blood pressure	High body-mass index	High fasting plasma glucose
4	Unsafe water	High fasting plasma glucose	High fasting plasma glucose	High blood pressure
5	Unsafe sanitation	Smoking	Particulate matter	Alcohol use

Data from Institute of Health Metrics and Evaluation (IHME). nd GBD Compare: Viz Hub. Retrieved from https://vizhub.healthdata.org/gbd-compare/

Demography and Health

There are a number of **demographic** matters that are extremely important to people's health. Among the most important are population growth, population aging, urbanization, the demographic divide, and the demographic transition.

Population Growth

The population of the world was estimated in 2019 to be about 7.7 billion. It is estimated that the world's population will be 9.7 billion in 2050.[19] The overwhelming majority of population growth in the future will occur in low- and middle-income countries, especially in sub-Saharan Africa. This reflects the fact that fertility is falling slowly in many countries that have had high fertility rates historically, whereas many of the high-income countries already have very low fertility. In fact, some high-income countries are below **replacement fertility**. At a minimum, we should expect that increasing population growth in low-income countries will put substantial pressure on the environment, with its attendant risks for health. It will also mean that infrastructure, such as water supply and sanitation, will have to be provided to an increasing number of people in the countries that have the largest service gaps and can least afford to expand such services. Increasing population size will also make it more difficult for low-income countries to provide education and health services. This could cause these countries to face substantial impacts on health as a result.

Population Aging

The population of the world is aging, especially in high-income countries that have low fertility. One impact of population aging is that it changes the ratio between the number of people who are 15 to 64 years of age compared with the number who are 65 years of age or older. This is called the **age dependency ratio**. In Niger, with high fertility and a growing population, only 5% of the population in 2019 was over 65 years of age. By contrast, in Japan, with very low fertility and a shrinking population, 47% of the population was over 65 in 2019.[20]

Population aging and the shift in the elderly support ratio have profound implications for the burden of disease and for health expenditures and how they will be financed. In the simplest terms, people will live longer and experience more years with morbidities and disabilities, largely related to noncommunicable diseases. This will raise the costs of health care. In addition, the large numbers of older adults for every working person will make it difficult for countries to finance that health care.

Urbanization

In the last 15 years, the majority of the world's population has lived in urban areas for the first time in world history. People are continuing to move from rural to urban areas, especially in low- and middle-income countries. Continuing urbanization will put enormous pressure on urban infrastructure, such as water and sanitation, schools, and health services, which are already in short supply in many countries. Gaps in infrastructure, as well as the development of crowded and low-standard housing, for example, could have substantial negative consequences for health.

The Demographic Transition

One important demographic trend of importance is called the **demographic transition**. Simply put, this is the shift from a pattern of high fertility and high mortality to low fertility and low mortality, with population growth occurring in between.[21]

When we look back historically at the countries that are now high-income, we can see that they had long periods when fertility was high, mortality was high, and population growth was, therefore, relatively slow, or might even have declined in the face of epidemics. Beginning around the turn of the 19th century, however, mortality in those countries began to decline as hygiene and nutrition improved and the burden of infectious diseases lessened. In most cases, this decline in mortality started before the deep decline in fertility. As mortality declined, the population increased, and the share of the population of younger ages also increased. Later, fertility began to decline and, as births and deaths became more equal, population growth slowed. As births and deaths stayed more equal, the share of the population that was of older ages increased. There are now some countries, as mentioned earlier, in which death rates exceed birth rates, and the population is declining. These populations, such as Italy, have the highest ratio of people over 65 to the rest of the population.

The Epidemiologic Transition

The **epidemiologic transition**[22] is closely related to the demographic transition. Historically, there has been a shift in the patterns of disease that follow these trends: first, high and fluctuating mortality, related to very poor health conditions, epidemics, and famine. Then, progressive declines in mortality as epidemics became less frequent. Finally, further declines in mortality, increases in life expectancy, and the predominance of noncommunicable diseases.

The pace of the epidemiologic transition in different societies depends on a number of factors related to the determinants of health. In its early stages, the transition appears to depend primarily on improvements in hygiene, nutrition, education, and socioeconomic status. Some improvements also stem from advances in public health and in medicine, such as the development of new vaccines and antibiotics.[23]

Discussion Questions

1. What is measured with the neonatal, infant, and child mortality rates? The maternal mortality ratio? Why is the latter over 100,000 live births, rather than over 1,000 live births, like the other indicators?
2. Which two World Bank regions have the worst health status indicators? Why?
3. What is a DALY? What value is gained by measuring the burden of disease in DALYs rather than in deaths?
4. What are the leading causes of adult death globally? Why is it important to know about this?
5. What are the most important risk factors in low-income countries for the death of children below 5 years of age?

References

1. The World Bank. Data. Mortality rate, under-5 (per 1,000 live births). nd, A. Retrieved from https://data.worldbank.org/indicator/SH.DYN.MORT?end=2019&start=2019
2. World Health Organization. *Determinants of health*. 2017. Retrieved from https://www.who.int/news-room/q-a-detail/determinants-of-health
3. World Health Organization. *Social determinants of health*. nd. Retrieved from http://www.who.int/social_determinants/sdh_definition/en/
4. The World Bank. Repositioning nutrition as central to development—A strategy for large-scale action. Washington, DC: World Bank; 2013.
5. Shonkoff JP, Garner AS. The lifelong effects of early childhood adversity and toxic stress. *Pediatrics (Evanston)*. 2012;129(1):e232-e246. https://doi.org/10.1542/peds.2011-2663
6. Basch P. *Textbook of international health* 2nd ed. New York, NY: Oxford University Press; 2001.
7. The World Bank. Data. Life expectancy at birth, total, (years). nd, B. Retrieved from https://data.worldbank.org/indicator/SP.DYN.LE00.IN
8. The World Bank. Data. Maternal Mortality Ratio (modeled estimate, per 100,000 live births). nd, C. Retrieved from: https://data.worldbank.org/indicator/SH.STA.MMRT
9. The World Bank. Data: Mortality rate, infant (per 1,000 live births). nd, D. Retrieved from https://data.worldbank.org/indicator/SP.DYN.IMRT.IN
10. The World Bank. Data. Mortality rate, neonatal (per 1,000 live births). nd, E. Retrieved from https://data.worldbank.org/indicator/SH.DYN.NMRT
11. Last JM. *A dictionary of epidemiology*. 4th ed. New York, NY: Oxford University Press; 2001.

12. Haupt A, Kane TT. *Population Reference Bureau's Population handbook*. 4th International edition. Population Reference Bureau; Washington, D. C.: 2000.

13. The World Bank. Data: Incidence of tuberculosis (per 100,000 people). nd, F. Retrieved from https://data.worldbank.org/indicator/SH.TBS.INCD

14. Institute of Health Metrics and Evaluation (IHME). GBD Compare: Viz Hub. nd, A. Retrieved from https://vizhub.healthdata.org/gbd-compare/

15. Lopez AD, Mathers CD, Murray CJL. The burden of disease and mortality by condition: data, methods, and results for 2001. In: AD Lopez, CD Mathers, M Ezzati, DT Jamison, CJL Murray, eds. *Global Burden of Disease and Risk Factors*. (pp. 45–240). New York, NY: Oxford University Press; 2006.

16. GBD 2016 Collaborators. The Global Burden of Disease Study 2016. *Lancet* 2017A; 390(10100):1083–1464. Retrieved from https://www.thelancet.com/journals/lancet/issue/vol390no10100/PIIS0140-6736(17)X0041-X

17. Institute of Health Metrics and Evaluation (IHME). IHME|GHDx|GBD Compare. *Global Burden of Disease Study 2019 (GBD 2019) Disability Weights*. nd, B. Retrieved from http://ghdx.healthdata.org/record/ihme-data/gbd-2019-disability-weights

18. The Lancet. *Global Burden of Disease*. 2020. Available at: https://www.thelancet.com/gbd #2019GBDIssue. https://www.thelancet.com/journals/lancet/issue/vol396no10258/PIIS0140 -6736(20)X0042-0

19. United Nations. *World Population Prospects 2019*. 2019. Retrieved from: https://population.un.org/wpp/Publications/Files/WPP2019_Highlights.pdf

20. The World Bank. Data: Age dependency ratio, old (% of working age population). nd. Retrieved from https://data.worldbank.org/indicator/SP.POP.DPND.OL

21. Lee R. The demographic transition: three centuries of fundamental change. *J Economic Perspect*. 2003;17(4):167–190.

22. Omran AR. The epidemiologic transition: a theory of the epidemiology of population change. *Milbank Quarterly*. 2005;83(4):731–757.

23. Jamison DT. Investing in health. In: Jamison DT, Breman JG, Meashem AR, et al. (Eds.) *Disease Control Priorities in Developing Countries*. New York, NY; Oxford University Press: 2006;3–34.

CHAPTER 3

Health Systems and Universal Health Coverage

LEARNING OBJECTIVES

By the end of this chapter, the reader will be able to do the following:

- Describe the main functions of a health system
- Review how health systems are organized
- Outline key health system issues and how they might be addressed
- Note the main features of universal health coverage (UHC) and measures that low- and lower middle-income countries can take to achieve UHC over time

VIGNETTES

Uchenna lived in Nigeria. She had a high fever and suspected she had malaria. Her family took her to the local health clinic. When they arrived, the community health worker who staffed the clinic was nowhere to be found. Uchenna's family knew that the clinic rarely operated as it was supposed to, so they took her to the district hospital. She waited 6 hours to be seen but was finally examined by a doctor and given medicine for malaria. Happily, she had a full recovery.

Cesar lived in San José, the capital of Costa Rica, and had been ill for some time. He visited his local health center, where he was referred to the national hospital because it appeared that he might have cancer. The hospital confirmed the diagnosis of cancer and then treated him with drugs and surgery. He stayed several weeks in the hospital during his recovery. The national health insurance program of Costa Rica covered the cost of Cesar's care. His cancer was detected early and treated appropriately, and 10 years later Cesar remains cancer free.

Introduction

This chapter is about health systems and the aim of attaining **universal health coverage (UHC)**.

When reading this chapter, it is important to keep in mind the following questions:

- To what extent do different health systems value the "right to health"?
- What is the extent to which universal health coverage has been achieved?
- What is the role in various health systems of individuals, and of the public and private sectors and of nongovernmental organizations (NGOs)?
- What is the extent to which different actors in the system are engaged in the financing and provision of health services?
- How are different health systems organized and managed?
- What are key issues constraining the effectiveness and efficiency of health systems in different settings?
- How can those constraints be addressed most effectively?

Some key terms that will be used are shown in **Table 3-1**.

Table 3-1 Definitions of Key Terms

Term	Definition
Health System Organization and Management	
Brain Drain	The migration of health personnel in search of a better standard of living and quality of life, higher salaries, access to advanced technology, and more stable political conditions in different places worldwide.
Governance	The actions and means adopted by a society to organize itself in the promotion and protection of the health of its population.
Health System	The sum of organizations, institutions, and resources whose primary purpose is to improve health.
Primary Care	The provision of first contact, person-focused, ongoing care over time that meets the health-related needs of people, refers (to a hospital) only those problems too uncommon to maintain competence, and coordinates care when people receive services at other levels of care.
Responsiveness to the Expectations of the Population	How the system performs relative to non-health aspects; meeting or not meeting a population's expectations of how it should be treated by providers of prevention, care, or nonpersonal services.
Secondary Care	Medical care provided by a specialist or facility upon referral by a primary care physician.

(continues)

Table 3-1 Definitions of Key Terms *(continued)*

Term	Definition
Health System Organization and Management	
Stewardship	The wide range of functions carried out by governments as they seek to achieve national health policy objectives.
Task Shifting	The rational redistribution of tasks among health workforce teams. Specific tasks are moved, where appropriate, from highly qualified health workers to health workers with shorter training and fewer qualifications to make more efficient use of the available human resources for health.
Tertiary Care	Specialized consultative care, usually on referral from primary or secondary medical care personnel, by specialists working in a center that has personnel and facilities for special investigation and treatment.
Financing Health Systems	
Conditional Cash Transfers	Programs that provide cash payments to poor households that meet certain behavioral requirements, generally related to children's health care and education.
Contracting In (Health Services)	One level of government or a public institution that contracts with a lower level of government facility, such as a district, a province, or another facility, to deliver services.
Contracting Out (Health Services)	A financing agency (government, insurance entity, or development partner), also known as a "purchaser," that provides resources to a nonstate provider (NSP, such as a nongovernmental organization [NGO] or private sector firm), also known as a "contractor," to provide a specified set of services, in a specified location, with specified objectives.
Fairness of Financial Contribution	The risks each household faces due to the costs of the health system are distributed according to ability to pay rather than to the risk of illness.
Financial Protection	Financing health care in a way that does not cause people to be denied access to health care or to become impoverished because of their inability to pay for health services.
Out-of-Pocket Health Expenditure	Any direct outlay by households, including gratuities and in-kind payments, to health practitioners and suppliers of pharmaceuticals, therapeutic appliances, and other goods and services whose primary intent is to contribute to the restoration or enhancement of the health status of individuals or population groups. It is a part of private health expenditure.
Private Health Expenditure	The sum of total expenditure on health by private entities, notably commercial insurance, nonprofit institutions, and households, including out-of-pocket health expenditures, patient copayments, private health insurance premiums, and health expenditures by nongovernmental organizations.

Public Health Expenditure	The sum of outlays by government entities to purchase healthcare services and goods, notably by ministries of health and social security agencies. The revenue base may comprise multiple sources, including external funds.
Results-Based Financing	Any program that rewards the delivery of one or more outputs or outcomes by one or more incentives, financial or otherwise, after the principal has verified that the agent has delivered the agreed-upon results.
Right to Health	The highest attainable standard of health is a fundamental right of every human being, including access to timely, acceptable, and affordable health care of appropriate quality.
Risk-pooling	Those who are healthy subsidize those who are sick, and those who are rich subsidize those who are poor.
Total Expenditure on Health	The sum of general government expenditure on health (commonly called public expenditure on health) and private expenditure on health.
Universal Health Coverage	Ensuring that all people can use the promotive, preventive, curative, rehabilitative, and palliative health services they need, of sufficient quality to be effective, while also ensuring that the use of these services does not expose the user to financial hardship.
User Fees	Charges levied at the point of use for any aspect of health services. For example, registration fees, consultation fees, fees for drugs and medical supplies, or charges for any health service rendered, such as outpatient or inpatient care.

What Is a Health System?

The World Health Organization (WHO) defines a **health system** as "the sum total of all the organizations, institutions and resources whose primary purpose is to improve health."[1]

The Functions of a Health System

The *World Health Report 2000*, produced by WHO, was about making health systems more effective and efficient. That report has been the basis for considerable analysis of the goals of health systems, their functions, how they are organized, and how well they perform. This report suggests that there are three goals for every health system: good health, responsiveness to the expectations of the population, and fairness of financial contribution.[2]

The report further suggests that each health system has four functions to play:[2] provide health services; raise money that can be spent on health, referred to as "resource generation"; pay for health services, referred to as "financing"; and govern and regulate the health system, referred to as "stewardship."

Elaborating somewhat on those ideas, one could say that all health systems should do the following:[3]

- Provide access to a comprehensive range of health services, including prevention, diagnosis, treatment, and rehabilitation
- Protect the sick and their families against the financial costs of ill health and disability through the establishment and operation of some type of insurance scheme
- Improve the health of populations through appropriate governance of the health system, regulation of that system, promotion of good health, and the carrying out of key public health functions, such as surveillance, the operation of public health laboratories, and food and drug regulation

WHO has also developed a framework for considering the different parts of health systems and the roles they play in health system performance.[4] This framework includes the six building blocks of a health system: service delivery; health workforce; information; medical products, vaccines, and technologies; financing; and leadership/governance.

The WHO framework suggests that if countries combine these building blocks with attention to ensuring quality, safety, and universality of coverage, services are most likely to improve health in equitable ways that are responsive to the needs of individuals, protect them from financial risk, and get as much health as possible for the money spent.

How Are Health Services Organized?

Categorizing Health Services

The manner in which health systems are organized is related to the history, politics, and values of individual countries. Countries generally spend more money per capita on health as their incomes rise. As countries become better-off, they usually focus greater attention on trying to ensure universal access to a basic package of health services and universal coverage of health insurance. As they develop economically, they also pay increasing attention to improving the quality, effectiveness, efficiency, and fairness of their health systems. Of course, one goal of low- and middle-income countries must be to address these aims, to the greatest extent possible, even before their incomes have risen.

There is no ideal way of categorizing healthcare systems because they are so varied and so complex. However, **Table 3-2** reflects one way of thinking about how health systems are organized.[5] Nonetheless, keep in mind that the table represents a dramatic oversimplification of a very complicated subject.

In Table 3-2 health systems are organized into three types:

- Some systems are organized around a national health service. In this approach, outside of a relatively small private health sector, the government is the sole payer for health care and owns most of the healthcare facilities.
- Other systems operate through a national health insurance scheme, such as in Canada, France, Germany, and Japan. These systems, in principle, offer health insurance to all people for an agreed package of services. People often refer to such systems as having "social health insurance."

- Pluralistic systems, such as those in the United States, India, and Nigeria, are those systems in which the public sector; private, for-profit sector; and private, not-for-profit sectors all play important roles.

Most low-income countries have a pluralistic health system that includes a publicly supported and provided health system and a range of private providers and facilities. They often have publicly organized insurance programs for government employees and relatively small private insurance markets. They may also have a number of community-based insurance schemes. Private out-of-pocket payments represent a substantial share of the costs of health care in countries that lack widespread insurance programs.

Many of the middle-income countries, particularly in Latin America, have organized a substantial part of their health system around a social health insurance

Table 3-2 Simplified Categorization of Approaches to Selected Health System Issues

	National Health Service	National Health Insurance	Pluralistic
Health as a Right	Fundamental	Fundamental	Health as a personal good
Ownership of Facilities	Overwhelmingly public	Vast majority public and private, not-for-profit	Public, private, for-profit and private, not-for-profit
Employment of Providers	The health service and private	Largely private	Largely private
Form of Insurance	Overwhelmingly public insurance linked to the health service	Largely government single payers and firms working with government schemes	Public insurance; private, for-profit insurance, and private, not-for-profit insurance, with substantial numbers lacking insurance
Financing of Insurance	Overwhelmingly tax-based	Some based on individual premiums, others based on employee and employer payroll taxes, and some are tax-based	Taxes, employer and employee insurance contributions, individual purchase of insurance, and out-of-pocket
Country Examples	United Kingdom, Cuba	France, Canada, Japan, Germany, Brazil, Mexico, Thailand	India, Nigeria, United States

Data from Birn A-E, Pillay Y, & Holtz TH (2009). *Textbook of international health.* New York, NY: Oxford University Press.

scheme or schemes. Many of them are also working to better coordinate and expand the schemes to be universal in coverage. Private out-of-pocket expenditures are generally lower in these countries than in many other low- and middle-income countries and are concentrated on those individuals who are not covered by the insurance schemes.

It is important to keep the concepts of *financing* and *provision* of healthcare services conceptually separate, and then to examine the extent to which the public and private sector deliver healthcare services in settings with varying financing arrangements.

Levels of Care

Health systems are generally organized into three levels of care: primary, secondary, and tertiary. In most high-income countries, primary care is provided by a physician, who is the first point of contact with the patient. Secondary care is usually provided by physicians and general hospitals, which are often located in towns and cities. Tertiary care is provided in specialized hospitals that are generally located only in cities.

Many low- and middle-income countries have established primary, secondary, and tertiary-level facilities by geographic area, depending on the size of the population. These countries, for example, might have a center for primary care for every 5,000 to 10,000 people, a secondary hospital in each district, and a tertiary hospital in large cities. In many low-income countries, medical assistants, nurses, or nurse-midwives would staff the lowest level of the system. The first level at which there might be a trained physician would be in large primary healthcare centers or district hospitals.

Primary Health Care from Alma-Ata to the Present

One of the historic and core ideas about health systems is the notion of "primary health care," which springs partly from a historic conference in 1978 in Alma-Ata (now called Almaty) in Kazakhstan in the former Soviet Union. This was one of the most important meetings in the history of global health, and it produced the Declaration of Alma-Ata.[6] The notion of primary health care that was articulated at Alma-Ata remains an important one. Many countries, at all income levels, continue to work toward a model of primary health care that is effective and efficient and grounded in the community.

The Roles of the Public, Private, and NGO Sectors

It is important to distinguish among the different actors that participate in health systems and the different functions they serve. The public sector is the first actor in most health systems. The involvement of the public sector could be at the national, state, or municipal level, depending on the country. The public sector is responsible for the stewardship of the system, meaning its governance, policy setting, rulemaking, and enforcement of rules. The public sector is also responsible for raising the funds for the health system, making decisions about allocating those funds, and establishing approaches to health insurance. In addition, the public sector is responsible for managing and financing key public health functions, such as setting public health policies, enforcing laws related to health, disease surveillance, and food and drug regulations. In some countries, the public sector provides health services through facilities that it owns and operates. However, the public sector can also purchase health services from the private for-profit or private not-for-profit sectors.

Although some people believe that health is a right that should not be "for sale," the private for-profit sector is involved in the provision and financing of health systems in all countries. There are many types of private health service providers that go beyond those involved in formal health services. Especially in low- and middle-income countries, people often buy health services from a range of unlicensed medical practitioners, such as medicine men, shamans, healers, bonesetters and traditional birth attendants. Many people also seek care from practitioners of traditional forms of medicine, such as those in China and India. In addition, people often get medical advice from drug vendors who operate small kiosks or mobile drug stores, or from pharmacies and pharmacists. In high-income countries, too, people make use of a wide range of health practitioners.

When one thinks about the private not-for-profit sector, particularly in low- and middle-income countries, one is often thinking about **nongovernmental organizations (NGOs)**. Broadly defined, an NGO is:

> A not-for-profit, voluntary citizens' group, which is organized on a local, national, or international level to address issues in support of the public good. Some are organized around specific issues, such as human rights.[7]

NGOs may be large or small; may be local, national, or international; and may work in one or many areas of activity. NGOs are actively involved in many areas of health in many countries. Typical examples would be in community-based efforts to promote better health through health education and improved water supply and sanitation. NGOs are also very involved in carrying out various health services. Like the private for-profit sector, NGOs can operate with their own financing, or they can work under contract to the government, the private sector, or the philanthropic sector.

A critical issue in designing and operating health systems is the roles that ought to be assigned to the public, private for-profit, private not-for-profit, and NGO sectors and how those roles should be paid for. It is particularly important to carefully consider the extent to which the public sector should provide services, compared with the extent to which it would be more cost-efficient for the public sector to buy certain services from the private for-profit and private not-for-profit sectors. It could be the case that public sector health services at the primary level are not as effective and efficient as similar services operated by the NGO sector.

Health System Expenditure

The health sector is an important part of the economy in all countries and a matter on which governments and private individuals spend a substantial amount of resources. Total health expenditure as a share of GDP varies substantially across countries. It is around 2 to 4% in a number of countries, such as Indonesia, Pakistan, and Nigeria. Several low- and middle-income countries spend about 4 to 7% of their GDP on health. Most of the higher-income countries spend between 8 and 12% of their GDP on health. However, the United States spends almost 17% of its GDP on health. In addition, there are some countries that spend a substantially higher share of GDP on health than one might anticipate given their income level, including Afghanistan, Brazil, Costa Rica, and Cuba.[8]

We can also see a very wide range in the share of total expenditure on health that is attributable to the private sector. Only about 15 to 25% of total expenditure on health is private-sector expenditure in a number of high-income countries that have substantial health insurance programs, such as Denmark and France. In some other high-income countries, such as Ireland and Israel, private-sector expenditure as a share of total expenditure on health is between 35 and 40%. On the other hand, in a number of low- and lower middle-income countries, such as India, Nepal, Nigeria, and Pakistan, which lack widespread coverage with formal insurance, private sector expenditure on health as a share of total expenditure on health is approximately 60 to 75%.[9]

It is valuable when examining data on health expenditure to compare it with health outcomes. Thailand, for example, has managed to achieve relatively good health with a relatively low level of expenditures and low out-of-pocket costs. This raises important questions about how other countries might do the same. Countries spend more per capita on health as their incomes rise. This is, in part, because when they have more to spend, they face a greater burden of noncommunicable diseases, and the popular demands on their systems are significant. In fact, the average per capita spending on health annually is as follows:[8] low-income: $36; lower middle-income: $86; upper middle-income: $486; and high-income: $5,562.

Levels of expenditure, both as a share of GDP and per capita, however, need to be considered for their effectiveness and efficiency. The goal of a country is not to spend high sums on health; rather, it is to enable the best health of its people at least cost, in doable, sustainable, and fairly distributed ways.

The Quest for Universal Health Coverage

As noted earlier, the goal of a health system should be the attainment of universal health coverage, in as cost-efficient a manner as possible, in fairly distributed ways, with particular attention to the marginalized members of society. According to WHO, the aim of universal health coverage is to ensure that people get the health services they need, when and where they need them, and without suffering financial hardship when paying for them. WHO also suggests that this aim reflects three fundamental concerns: fairness of access to services, regardless of people's ability to pay for them; appropriate quality of services; and financial arrangements for services that protect people from suffering financial hardship.[10]

In principle, the achievement of universal health coverage requires, first of all, a health system that works. Building on the WHO health systems framework described earlier in the chapter, this would ideally mean a system that has the following components:[11]

- Offers an integrated package of basic services for maternal and child health, noncommunicable diseases, and the control of key communicable diseases, such as HIV, TB, malaria, and neglected tropical diseases (NTDs)
- Is affordable
- Offers fair access to essential medicine and medical technologies
- Has a well-trained and highly motivated workforce

Of course, these inputs must also be managed effectively if a health system is to function properly and achieve desired outcomes at a reasonable cost.

Although countries can provide financial protection in a number of ways, most have chosen to do so by pooling risks across part or all of the population through insurance. As countries seek to develop an insurance scheme, they face a number of key questions, such as:[12] Who should be covered? What services should be covered? What share of the costs should the insurance scheme pay?

Countries, especially low-income ones, must also wrestle with how they will finance the provision of insurance. Generally, countries may finance insurance through some combination of payroll taxes on employers and employees, general taxes, and contributions from the insured in the form of premiums.[12]

As countries establish programs for UHC, they must also assess the most efficient and effective ways to pay the healthcare providers from whom the insurance system will buy services. Should this be on a fee-for-service basis, a fixed fee per person covered per year (capitation), paying for the achievement of certain health goals, or the successful completion of certain procedures?[12]

Countries must also wrestle with questions concerning how they will organize their risk-pooling (insurance) arrangements. Should they have a single national insurance scheme, many schemes operated by different groups, or many schemes based on different kinds of beneficiaries?[12]

The operation of insurance schemes requires careful attention to deciding how those schemes will finance the purchase of services. Should insurance cover the costs of public sector services, private sector services, or both? Will it be fair, effective, or efficient if the public sector continues to offer free or nearly free but often low-quality services to mostly poor people, whereas other people are able to purchase insurance and buy services that are often of higher quality in the private sector?[12,13]

For many years, there was enormous skepticism about the possibility that some countries, especially low-income ones, could achieve universal health coverage. Today, however, there is a global movement around ensuring that all countries achieve UHC as rapidly as possible. In fact, there have been a number of countries that have made important progress toward achieving UHC, including some countries that continue to have very low per capita income.[13–17]

Moving toward UHC is a highly political matter and achieving it will not come quickly or easily in most settings. This suggests that many countries may wish to take a phased approach, such as Mexico did, by incrementally increasing the coverage of both more people and more services.[16]

Learning from Health Systems Globally

Much can be learned from examining health systems in a number of countries, across all country income groups. However, space does not allow such an examination here. Readers are, therefore, encouraged to explore the health systems, for example, in France, Germany, and the United Kingdom; Costa Rica and Brazil; China and India; and Ghana and Rwanda.

Key Health System Issues

Considering the WHO criteria for measuring health system performance, it is clear that some health systems produce better outcomes than others. Health systems in high-income countries, for example, produce better results than the systems in low-income countries. The systems in high-income countries are typically better organized and managed, have greater financial resources, and have better trained and more abundant human resources for health. Almost all high-income countries have also had universal health coverage for many years, with substantial amounts of financial protection linked to it. By contrast, the health systems of the poorest countries are likely to have substantial managerial issues, lack financial and human resources, and have large gaps in the achievement of universal coverage. They also suffer substantial issues related to the quality of care.

Nonetheless, even countries that are resource poor can achieve good health outcomes if they are committed to the health of their people, make cost-efficient and fair choices about the policies that should lead the health sector, manage that sector with rigor, and also invest in addressing the determinants of health in effective and efficient ways. Costa Rica, Cuba, and China, for example, were able to substantially enhance the health of their people, even when they had relatively low levels of income.

As we explore health systems in greater detail, it is clear that all systems wrestle with a variety of challenges and constraints. These themes are explored briefly here.

Demographic and Epidemiologic Change

Except in countries in conflict and not counting the COVID-19 pandemic, people are living longer. As they do so, societies face higher burdens of noncommunicable diseases. Many of these conditions are chronic, and the cost of treating them is high compared with acute bouts of communicable diseases or conditions that occur at younger ages. As a result, relatively poor countries, with few resources to spend on health and weak institutions to address health issues, face a triple burden of disease simultaneously—the burdens of noncommunicable disease, communicable disease, and injuries.[18]

Stewardship

The quality of governance is an important determinant of outcomes in the health sector. In high-income countries, the health sector will tend to be governed in relatively effective, open, and transparent ways, with little corruption. Unfortunately, however, governance in many low- and middle-income settings will tend to be weak across most sectors, and governments in low- and middle-income countries are often unable to enforce health sector rules and regulations. This may be especially true with respect to the inability of the health sector to oversee the work of the private healthcare sector, the management of healthcare personnel, or procurement.[19]

Human Resource Issues

The most severe human resource issues in better-off countries tend to be imbalances in the number of certain types of healthcare personnel. This contributes to the problem of "brain drain" in the healthcare sector of low- and middle-income countries.[20] The human resource issues in many low-income countries are considerable. The very poorest countries, especially in sub-Saharan Africa, will not have enough healthcare personnel to operate a health system effectively. They will also face significant gaps in qualified health service managers, both clinical and nonclinical. In addition, the quality of training, knowledge, and skills of many of their healthcare staff will be deficient.

Quality of Care

The United States National Academy of Medicine (NAM) (formerly the Institute of Medicine (IOM)) defines quality as "the degree to which health services for individuals and populations increase the likelihood of desired health outcomes and are consistent with current professional knowledge." According to NAM, health services need to be safe, effective, patient centered, timely, efficient, and equitable.[21]

There is good evidence that many health systems suffer from important problems of quality, and that quality varies considerably within health systems. Studies in the United States, for example, showed that "physicians complied with evidence-based guidelines for at least 80% of patients in only 8 of 306 U.S. hospital regions."[22] In a study in Papua New Guinea, a low-income country with rampant malaria, only 24% of health workers could indicate the correct treatment for malaria.[23]

There are many causes of poor-quality health services in low- and middle-income countries, including poor management, a lack of financial resources, poorly trained and inappropriately deployed staff, a failure of staff to do their work as intended, and unempowered patients. Many health systems also provide very little supervision of healthcare personnel and have only weak systems for monitoring the performance of their health system.[22] It is important to remember that in the health sector, poor-quality services are not just a waste of money. Rather, there is a direct link between the poor quality of services and people's health and well-being.

The Financing of Health Systems

The health systems in many countries battle continually for sufficient financing to meet their highest priorities in effective and efficient ways. Many countries, especially better-off ones, face issues of rising costs because of aging populations and the ever-increasing demands for the use of new technologies and new drugs.

In addition, all health systems ration health services to some extent. In many high-income countries, a critical issue is how to find the funding that is needed, even with increased efficiency, to reduce the waiting times for certain medical procedures that are financed through the national insurance program. A few of the high-income countries, such as Switzerland and the United States, also face important questions about the share of their total GDP that they are devoting to health and the implications of this for the rest of the economy. As one might expect, the financing issue in most low- and middle-income countries often revolves around the absolute lack of public sector financial resources for health, as well as the efficiency and effectiveness of their use.

Financial Protection

The capacity of people to pay for health services is a barrier to their access to health care, and catastrophic health costs impoverish people in many settings. In most high-income countries, this is not a significant problem because they have social health insurance schemes and essentially offer health insurance to all of their people. However, the lack of financial protection is a common problem in poorer countries. An earlier study in India showed, for example, that expenditure on health was a leading cause of families falling below the poverty line and a major cause of families selling assets to pay their bills for health care.[24]

Access and Equity

Health disparities are an important feature of many health systems. In low- and middle-income countries, disparities in access to services and in equity are often reflected in the following ways, among others:

- A lack of coverage of basic health services in areas where poor, rural, and minority people live.
- Services with a lower level of inputs in the areas noted above compared with other areas, such as fewer trained personnel and less equipment and drugs.
- Better-off people getting access to relatively expensive services that are generally less available to lower-income and socially marginalized groups.

Addressing Key Health Sector Concerns

There are few easy answers to effectively address the most critical health sector issues, particularly in low-income countries. Nevertheless, there is an increasing body of evidence about measures that can be taken to deal with some of the problems noted previously and to design and manage health systems more effectively and efficiently. These are discussed briefly here.

Demographic and Epidemiologic Change

The very poorest countries can take only a limited number of steps at once to deal with the multiple burdens of communicable and noncommunicable diseases and injuries. Perhaps the single most important step that low- and middle-income countries can take today to reduce the future burden of cardiovascular disease is to reduce the disease burden that is related to tobacco use. There is very good evidence that even in low-income settings, measures to make it harder and more expensive to buy cigarettes can reduce tobacco smoking.[25] They can also take other measures to begin to reduce road traffic accidents, including better engineering of roads, safer cars, and more traffic enforcement.[26]

The way in which health systems are organized and operated in many low- and middle-income countries will also need to be strengthened to address the growing burden of noncommunicable diseases.[27]

Stewardship

It will also be difficult to improve health system governance in countries in which overall governance is weak and corruption is high. Nonetheless, a number of measures are proving to be useful in addressing key governance issues in health. Contracting out some services, carrying out customer satisfaction surveys among the users of the health system, and letting communities provide services with "citizen report cards" are also proving to be helpful to enhancing governance in some settings.[19]

Human Resources

The problems of human resources for health relate largely to a lack of staff, a maldistribution of staff, the inadequate training and quality of personnel, and the poor environment in which many of them carry out their work. An international group examining human resources for health highlighted the need for countries and their development partners to provide greater support for education and training of health personnel and to develop better policies and programs for retaining personnel.[28]

Even as they seek to address these problems in more comprehensive ways, some countries have taken steps to deal with human resource issues. Countries might be able to reduce the share of their health workers who are migrating, for example, by training them so they gain needed skills but do not get credentials for those skills that would be recognized by other countries.[29] Moreover, lower-level health personnel can be trained to carry out a number of functions often reserved for higher-level staff, a strategy known as **task shifting**. In Malawi, where there is an acute shortage of doctors, nurses were trained to perform caesarean sections.[29] A number of countries also use financial incentives to encourage better performance of healthcare personnel.[29]

Financing Health Services

The scope for very low-income countries to raise additional resources for health is limited, given the overall scarcity of resources. Nevertheless, there is some scope for shifting resources from other areas of the economy in some countries, given the potentially high returns to investments in health. Some of the low-income countries, however, will require development assistance for health for some time in order to boost expenditure on health and more effectively address some of their key health concerns, such as HIV/AIDS.[30]

There is also some scope for enhancing health outcomes by shifting expenditure within the health sector. By focusing expenditure on a selected group of low-cost investments that are known to be effective if managed properly, even very poor countries may be able to improve the health outcomes of their poorest people.[2,31]

Many countries also have substantial room for improving the efficiency of the resources they spend on health. WHO has estimated that between 20 and 40% of the expenditures on health in low-income countries are wasted by spending that is not effective or efficient.[4]

Financial Protection and Universal Coverage

Over the longer term, today's low- and middle-income countries aspire to having a health system that provides universal health coverage, coupled with a high degree of financial protection. We can think of this, for example, as their wanting to move as rapidly as possible toward having a system like that of France or the Netherlands—a system that covers all of the population for many health conditions with a generous insurance package and limited out-of-pocket payments.

A recent study defined a package of the highest priority investments that could be a starting point for the further development of UHC in low- and lower middle-income countries. This package would include key efforts to address outstanding Group I causes and the highest priority investments for noncommunicable diseases and injuries. As countries make progress in implementing this "highest-priority package," they could expand services that are part of their UHC scheme to an even broader package.[31]

Access and Equity

Many countries have not focused sufficient attention on the health of their disadvantaged people and have not been sufficiently aware of the kinds of gaps in health coverage and health status that these people face. Very substantial gains could be made in health status within many countries, for example, if the coverage of effective programs for at least childhood vaccination, TB, and malaria were increased among the poor.

Quality

There is good evidence that quality can be enhanced in a number of ways even in the absence of substantial additional resources.

The recent global commission on the quality of care suggested a number of broad measures that are essential to quality:[32]

- Governments must make quality the foundation of their systems.
- Governments and their citizens must ignite a demand for quality services.
- Services need to be redesigned to focus on quality outcomes rather than access alone.
- Countries should revise the training of providers to focus on competency-based training and providing better support for those workers.
- Health systems should measure and report on what matters most—outcomes, competent care, user experience, and confidence in the system.

Pharmaceuticals

Pharmaceuticals play a fundamental role in all health systems. Health systems and consumers also spend considerable sums on them. Countries need to be able to buy the right drugs at the best possible price and ensure that they are prescribed, dispensed, and used properly. The same is true, of course, for diagnostics and vaccines. Yet, there are major issues concerning the purchase of drugs that are not essential, that are of low quality, or that are counterfeit. There are also large issues around the appropriate use of all drugs, especially antibiotics. WHO has been extensively involved in major efforts at helping countries to specify lists of "essential drugs" and to procure drugs of acceptable quality at the best possible price. UNICEF has also been deeply involved with helping countries to procure pharmaceuticals.

Discussion Questions

1. What is a health system? What are its key functions?
2. What is the meaning of universal health coverage? Why is achieving it so important?
3. Discuss the most important differences between national health insurance systems, social health insurance systems, and pluralistic systems.
4. Discuss some of the most critical issues in the health systems in low-income countries and steps they might take to address them.
5. In what ways will demographic changes affect the demands on health systems in low- and middle-income countries over the next few decades?

References

1. World Health Organization (WHO). Q&As: health systems. nd. Retrieved from https://www.who.int/topics/health_systems/qa/en/
2. World Health Organization (WHO). *The world health report 2000.* Geneva, Switzerland: World Health Organization; 2000.
3. Southby, R. *Health System Organization.* Presented at George Washington University, Washington, DC; 2004.
4. World Health Organization (WHO). *Everybody's business: strengthening health systems to improve health outcomes: WHO's framework for action.* Geneva, Switzerland: World Health Organization; 2007.
5. Birn, A-E, Pillay, Y, & Holtz, TH. *Textbook of International Health.* New York, NY: Oxford University Press; 2009.
6. World Health Organization (WHO). *Declaration of Alma-Ata.* International Conference on Primary Health Care, September 6–12, 1978, Alma-Ata, USSR. Geneva, Switzerland; 1978.
7. United Nations Civil Society Unit. *United Nations: definitions and terms.* Retrieved from https://www.apa.org/international/united-nations/acronyms.pdf. nd.
8. World Bank. *Data. Current Health Expenditure (% of GDP).* nd, A. Retrieved from: https://data.worldbank.org/indicator/SH.XPD.CHEX.GD.ZS
9. World Bank. Data. Domestic private health expenditure (% of current health expenditure). nd, B. Retrieved from: https://data.worldbank.org/indicator/SH.XPD.PVTD.CH.ZS
10. World Health Organization (WHO). *Health financing for universal coverage.* Retrieved from http://www.who.int/health_financing/universal_coverage_definition/en/. 2014A
11. World Health Organization (WHO). *Universal health coverage.* Retrieved from http://www.who.int/features/qa/universal_health_coverage/en/. 2014B
12. World Health Organization (WHO). *World health report 2010.* Geneva, Switzerland; 2010.

13. Langomarsino G, Gabarant A, Adyas A, Muga R, Otoo N. Moving towards universal health coverage: health insurance reforms in nine developing countries in Africa and Asia. *Lancet.* 2012;380(9845):933–943.

14. Tangcharoensathien V, Patcharanarumol W, Ir P, et al. Health-financing reforms in southeast Asia: challenges in achieving universal coverage. *Lancet.* 2011;377(9768):863–873.

15. Kumar AKS, Chen LC, Choudhury M, et al. Financing health care for all: challenges and opportunities. *Lancet.* 2011;377(9766):668–679.

16. Atun, R, de Andrade LO, Almeida G, et al. Universal health coverage in Latin America 1—health-system reform and universal coverage in Latin America. *Lancet.* 2014;1–18. doi: 10.1016/S0140-6736(14)61646-9

17. Reich MR, Harris J, Ikegami N, et al. Moving towards universal health coverage: lessons from 11 country studies. *Lancet.* 2016;387(10020):811–816.

18. Mathers CD, Lopez AD, Murray CJL. The burden of disease and mortality by condition: data, methods, and results for 2001. In: Lopez AD, Mathers CD, Ezzati M, Jamison DT, Murray CJL, eds, *Global Burden of Disease and Risk Factors.* New York, NY: Oxford University Press; 2006: 45–93.

19. Lewis, M. *Tackling healthcare corruption and governance woes in developing countries* (Working Paper 78). Washington, DC: Center for Global Development; 2006.

20. Physicians for Human Rights. *An action plan to prevent brain drain: building equitable health systems in Africa.* Retrieved from http://physiciansforhumanrights.org/library/reports/action-plan-to-prevent-brain-drain-africa-2004.html. 2004

21. Institute of Medicine (IOM). *Measuring the quality of health care.* Washington, DC: Institute of Medicine; 1999.

22. Peabody JW, Taguiwalo MM, Robalino DA, Frenk J. Improving the quality of care in developing countries. In: Jamison DT, Breman JG, Measham AR, et al., eds. *Disease Control Priorities in Developing Countries.* 2nd edition. New York, NY: Oxford University Press; 2006: 1293–1307.

23. Beracochea E, Dickenson R, Freeman P, Thomason J. Case management quality assessment in rural areas of Papua New Guinea. *Tropical Doctor.* 1995;25(2):69–74.

24. Peters DH, Preker AS, Yazbek AS, et al. *Better health systems for India's poor.* Washington, DC: The World Bank; 2002.

25. Jha P, Chaloupka FJ, Moore J, et al. *Tobacco Addiction.* In: Jamison DT, Breman JG, Measham AR, et al., eds. *Disease Control Priorities in Developing Countries* 2nd edition. New York, NY: Oxford University Press; 2006: 869–885.

26. Norton R, Hyder AA, Bishai D, Peden M. Unintentional injuries. In: Jamison DT, Breman JG, Measham AR, et al., eds. *Disease Control Priorities in Developing Countries* 2nd edition. New York, NY: Oxford University Press; 2006: 737–753.

27. Samb B, Desai N, Nishtar S, et al. Prevention and management of chronic disease: a litmus test for health-systems strengthening in low-income and middle-income countries. *Lancet.* 2010;376(9754):1785–1797.

28. Joint Learning Initiative. *Human resources for health: overcoming the crisis.* Cambridge, MA: Joint Learning Initiative; 2004.

29. Hongoro C, Normand C. Health workers: building and motivating the workforce. In: Jamison DT, Breman JG, Measham AR, et al., eds. *Disease Control Priorities in Developing Countries.* 2nd edition. New York, NY: Oxford University Press; 2006:1309–1322.

30. Resch S, Ryckman T, Hecht R. Funding AIDS programmes in the era of shared responsibility: an analysis of domestic spending in 12 low-income and middle-income countries. *The Lancet Global Health.* 2015;3(1):e52–e61.

31. Jamison DT, Gelband H, Horton S, et al., eds. *Disease Control Priorities: Improving Health and Reducing Poverty.* 3rd edition. Washington, DC: The World Bank; 2018:9.

32. Kruk ME, Gage AD, Arsenault C, et al. High-quality health systems in the Sustainable Development Goals era: time for a revolution. *The Lancet Global Health.* 2018;6(11): e1196–e1252. doi: 10.1016/S2214-109X(18)30386-3

CHAPTER 4

Environmental and Occupational Health and Intersectoral Approaches

LEARNING OBJECTIVES

By the end of this chapter, the reader will be able to do the following:

- Discuss the most important environmental and occupational threats to health, especially for low- and middle-income countries
- Review the burden of disease related to environmental and occupational risks
- Comment on the costs and consequences of key environmental and occupational health burdens
- Describe some of the most cost-effective ways of reducing the global burden of environmental and occupational health problems
- Take a more holistic view of the factors that determine health and the range of measures across agencies that are needed to ensure better health

VIGNETTES

Sunisa is a young mother in a rural area in northern Laos. She has two daughters, aged 1 and 3. Sunisa is not wealthy. Her house has no water connection. Thus, she collects water daily from the stream about half a mile from her house in containers she carries on her head. She stores the containers at the edge of her house, covered by cloth. Sunisa had only a little formal education and did nothing to purify the water. Her two daughters regularly have bouts of diarrhea, partly the result of drinking unsafe water.

Shahnaz is a 24-year-old woman in Pakistan. She has been sick for some time with coughing, night sweats, and weight loss. She fears that she has tuberculosis (TB). However, she will not seek treatment for her illness for fear of being forced from her home by her husband's family if she is found to have TB. The crowded conditions in which she lives put her at risk for contracting TB. Gender norms in her country mitigate against her seeking and receiving appropriate care for TB. Can the ministry of health alone address these issues in the short or medium term? Or, will it need to work in tandem with agencies such as the ministry of education and the women's development program?

Environmental Health

The Importance of Environmental Health

Environmental health issues are major risk factors for the global burden of disease. One study, which took a broad view of environmental risk factors, concluded that 22% of global deaths and 23% of the global burden of disease are attributable to environmental risk factors.[1]

Key Environmental Health Terms

In some cases, the word *environment* is defined very broadly, meaning everything that is not genetic. In other cases, the word *environment* includes only physical, chemical, or biological agents that directly affect health. For the purposes of this chapter, the **environment** is largely defined as "external physical, chemical, and microbiological exposures and processes that impinge upon individuals and groups and are beyond the immediate control of individuals."[2]

It is also valuable to understand the meaning of **environmental health**. This generally refers to a set of public health efforts that "is concerned with preventing disease, death, and disability by reducing exposure to adverse environmental conditions and promoting behavior change."[3] Another term that is commonly used when speaking about environmental health is **WASH**. This refers to "water, sanitation, and hygiene."

In thinking about the environment and health, it is important to consider the key types of environmental risk, the setting and scale at which one is exposed to such risks, and how one might be exposed to them. In simple terms, we can think of microbiological, biological, and physical risks that occur at the following levels: the household, the workplace, the community, regionally, and globally. We are generally exposed to such risks through air, water, or food. Examples include diarrhea related to unsafe water and sanitation, vehicle emissions leading to respiratory diseases, and injury or death from exposure to extreme heat or cold.[4]

Key Environmental Health Burdens

Household Air Pollution from Solid Fuels

WHO estimates that approximately 3 billion people in the world depend on solid fuel for their cooking and heating. Such fuels include the fossil fuel coal and the biomass fuels of animal dung, wood, logging wastes, and crop waste.[5] In the cases that most concern us, cooking and heating are done on open stoves that are not vented to the outside. These are generally used by lower-income groups, because people usually move to kerosene or gas for cooking and switch to improved stoves and better ventilation as their family income grows.

Smoke from burning biomass inside the home can produce conjunctivitis, upper respiratory irritation, and acute respiratory infection. The carbon monoxide produced can lead to acute poisoning. Other gases and smoke are associated over the long term with cardiovascular disease, chronic obstructive pulmonary disease, adverse reproductive outcomes, and cancer.[6] Women and children are especially vulnerable to the effects of household air pollution.

Ambient Particulate Matter Pollution

Many pollutants can be found in the **ambient air**. The most common effects of ambient air pollution are respiratory symptoms, including cough, irritation of the nose and throat, and shortness of breath.[7] In addition, older and younger people are generally most susceptible to the health effects of ambient particulate matter pollution.

Water, Sanitation, and Hygiene

WHO estimated that in 2017, about 71% of the global population, or about 5.3 billion people, had access to "a safely managed drinking water service." This is defined as "one located on premises, available when needed, and free from contamination." WHO also estimated that about 1.4 billion people had access to only "basic service" for water. This is defined as "an improved drinking-water source within a round trip of 30 minutes to collect water." Another 206 million people were estimated to have had only "limited service," requiring more than 30 minutes to collect water. Unfortunately, about 144 million people still depend on surface water sources. Moreover, it is estimated that almost 2 billion people in the world depend on water sources that are contaminated with human waste.[8] In addition, access to safe water generally varies with country income level and the income levels of different regions within countries.

In fact, water-related infections are numerous in low- and middle-income countries and among the most important in terms of the burden of disease. These pathogens are associated with diarrhea and many other gastrointestinal problems. They can be deadly when they lead to severe diarrhea and dehydration. Such diseases are especially risky for the very young, the very old, and people who have compromised immune systems, such as people living with HIV/AIDS.

WHO estimated that in 2017, approximately 74% of the world's population, or about 5.5 billion people, had access to at least a basic sanitation service. Only about 45% of the people in the world used a safely managed sanitation service. Unfortunately, about 2.0 billion people had no sanitation facilities and almost 673 million people were still defecating in the open.[9] Access to improved sanitation also generally varies by country and regional income level.

There is good evidence that improved disposal of human waste is associated with reductions in diarrheal disease, intestinal parasites, and trachoma. Failure to dispose properly of human waste contaminates water and food sources and leads to an increase in transmission of pathogens through the oral–fecal route. Failure to improve sanitation is also associated with the spread of parasitic worms, such as ascaris and hookworm. Improved sanitation reduces the burden of trachoma, because the flies that are significantly involved in the spread of that disease often breed in human waste.[10]

One area of hygiene, handwashing with soap, is especially important for good health. Unfortunately however, there is little data about the rates of handwashing with soap, or even on the availability of soap and water at designated places, which is used as a proxy for handwashing. The best available data is from a sample of 78 countries throughout the world. North America and Europe showed consistently high rates of basic handwashing facilities. The five countries surveyed in East and Southeast Asia also showed rates between 65 and 90%. In Latin America, the rates varied from about 25 to over 90%, similar to the rates for western Asia and northern Africa. The rates in central Asia and southern Asia varied from only about 5% to almost universal facilities. In sub-Saharan Africa, the rates varied from about 0 to about 50%.[11]

The Burden of Environmentally Related Diseases

Household Air Pollution

Household air pollution was the ninth most important risk factor in 2019 for deaths globally, for both sexes and all ages. However, it was the most important risk factor in low-income countries and the seventh most important risk factor for lower middle-income countries.[12] WHO estimates that about 3.8 million people die yearly from exposure to household air pollution, including from pneumonia, stroke, ischemic heart disease, COPD, and lung cancer.[5]

Ambient Particulate Matter Pollution

In 2019, ambient particulate matter pollution was the fourth leading attributable risk factor for death globally. It was third in upper middle-income countries. It was the second leading attributable risk factor for death in lower middle-income countries.[12]

WHO estimates that ambient particulate matter pollution contributes to about 4.2 million deaths a year globally, including from lung cancer, acute lower respiratory infections, stroke, ischemic heart disease, and COPD. WHO also estimates that more than 90% of those deaths occur in low- and middle-income countries.[13] Children are especially susceptible to the effects of ambient particulate matter pollution, particularly at critical times in their early development. Cities are also disproportionately affected.[14]

Water, Sanitation, and Hygiene

Unsafe water was the 14th leading risk factor for deaths globally in 2019, but the fifth leading risk factor in low-income countries and the ninth leading risk factor in lower middle-income countries. The same study estimated that unsafe sanitation was the 22nd leading risk factor for deaths globally, but the eighth leading risk factor for low-income countries and the 13th for lower middle-income countries. No access to a handwashing facility was the 22nd leading risk factor globally, but the 10th leading risk factor in low-income countries and the 19th leading risk factor in lower middle-income countries.[12]

We should expect that the burden of disease related to these risk factors will fall disproportionately on children, who suffer a large share of the burden of disease from diarrhea. In fact, the *Global Burden of Disease Study 2019* estimated that unsafe water was the fourth leading risk factor for deaths of children under five years of age, unsafe sanitation was the fifth leading risk factor, and no access to handwashing was the sixth leading risk factor.[12]

Historical experiences in what are now the high-income countries and a number of studies in low- and middle-income countries suggest that improving water supply alone will not reduce diarrheal disease as needed. This seems to stem from the large share of diarrhea that is associated with food that is unsafe and with poor personal hygiene.[15] However, separate from any impact on the reduction of diarrheal disease, improvements in water supply are associated with important reductions in the burden of disease from dracunculiasis, schistosomiasis, and trachoma.[11]

The Costs and Consequences of Key Environmental Health Problems

The social and economic consequences of key environmental health issues are enormous. First, the fact that more than 20% of the total global burden of disease is due to environmental risk factors suggests substantial social and economic costs related to these issues.[16] Second, as indicated earlier, the burden of these risk factors and their related causes of disease fall disproportionately on poorer people. Third, these environmental health burdens have very negative consequences on productivity. The consequences of household air pollution, for example, are very costly to women and thus their families in terms of morbidity, disability, and days of reduced productivity from both acute and chronic illnesses. Young children are especially at risk from all three environmental issues discussed in this chapter. In addition, the elderly face particular risks from this pollution, which can exacerbate chronic health problems they already have, leading to additional disability and its attendant reduction in productivity.

Reducing the Burden of Disease

The next section examines some key measures for addressing the burden of environmental health issues.

Ambient Particulate Matter Pollution

The limited studies that have been done, mostly on high-income countries, suggest that low- and middle-income countries could take a number of cost-effective steps to reduce the health burden of ambient air pollution.[17] These can be in the domains of law, policy, regulation, and technology. Estimates suggest that such measures are a "good buy," with a $30 return on average for every dollar spent on pollution control.[14]

The following are some of the first measures that a number of large cities in low- and middle-income countries have taken to reduce ambient particulate matter pollution[17]: the introduction of unleaded gasoline, low-smoke lubricant for two-stroke engines, the banning of two-stroke engines, shifting to natural gas to fuel public vehicles, tightening emissions inspections on vehicles, and reducing the burning of garbage.

It would also be reasonable to ensure that governments in low- and middle-income countries use their regulatory authority to incorporate information about ambient particulate matter pollution in their policies on transportation and industrial development.[17]

Household Air Pollution from Solid Fuels

There are a number of areas in which actions could be taken to reduce household air pollution from the burning of solid fuels for cooking and heating. In terms of the source of pollution, cooking devices can be improved, less polluting fuels can be used, and families can reduce their need for these fuels by using solar cooking and heating. Some changes can also be made to the living environment. Mechanisms for venting smoke can be built into the house, for example, or the kitchen can be moved away from the main part of the house. People can also change their behaviors to reduce pollution or exposure to it by using dried fuels, properly maintaining their stoves and chimneys, and keeping children away from the cooking area.[18]

Public policy can also play a helpful role in trying to reduce household air pollution. The public sector, for example, can promote information and education about such pollution and how to reduce it in schools, in the media, and in communities. The government can also use tax policy to reduce the cost of cooking appliances and fuels that will reduce this pollution. If necessary, it could subsidize the cost of improved fuels and appliances for those below a certain income level. Governments could also undertake surveillance of the problem and, if possible, set and enforce standards for household air pollution, although this will certainly be beyond the capacity of many low-income countries.[18]

Sanitation

There are a number of different levels of technology associated with excreta disposal, many different forms of toilets, and a wide array of costs associated with them. Sanitation could range from the simple technology of bucket latrines to modern urban sewage systems. Although we usually think of toilets as owned by individuals, they can also be public and shared by many individuals and families.

The cost per person for methods of sanitary removal of human waste varies considerably. At the bottom levels of service, it appears that pour-flush latrines, ventilation-improved latrines, and simple pit latrines can be constructed in low- and middle-income settings for about $60. Assuming that these last approximately five years, the annual cost per capita would be about $12. The construction cost of conventional sewage systems in some countries is more than 10 times that amount. In addition, they need water to function properly, and water is often in short supply.[11] Work is ongoing to develop more cost-effective toilets, and in Bangladesh, a simple pour-flush pan has been developed that costs only about $0.27 per household to construct.[10] Contrary to what we might believe, all of these systems can be operated in a hygienic manner that addresses health concerns.[15]

Given the relatively low cost of simple methods of sanitation and their relative effectiveness, it might be surprising that such a small share of households in low- and middle-income countries have a sanitary means of excreta disposal. Yet, besides the cultural constraints to their use, there are some other important constraints as well:[10] lack of knowledge of options, lack of income to pay for the toilets, the lack of skills needed for construction, and constraints of local laws.

In some countries, the public sector leads the effort to build low-cost sanitation systems. The public sector may also subsidize the cost of toilets for the poorest families, given that these sanitation improvements provide benefits to society as a whole. In addition, the public sector can try to enforce regulations to require the use of toilets.[10] It is also possible, if the private sector believes that there is a market for low-cost sanitation, for such efforts to be handled in the private sector.[10] Promotion of improved sanitation can also be done with a public–private partnership and led by nongovernmental organizations (NGOs).[19]

The largest impact of improved sanitation is in the reduction of diarrhea. Some studies[16] suggest that improved sanitation facilities in low- and middle-income countries result in an average reduction in cases of diarrhea by 28%. It is very important to note that having a toilet seems to also increase the handwashing habits of families, which itself brings benefits, as discussed later.

Finally, the benefits of sanitary excreta removal go beyond reducing diarrhea. Improving sanitation should reduce the prevalence of several worms, including ascaris, trichuris, and hookworm.[10] Given the low cost of some forms of latrines, they would be cost-effective approaches to reducing the prevalence of these worms. As noted earlier, the same would be true in terms of the positive impact and low costs of reducing trachoma through improved sanitation.[20]

Water Supply

There are many analogies between water supply and sanitation. For water, as well as for sanitation, there are many different levels of technology, and costs vary considerably according to the level of technology employed. One could get water, for example, from the following types of improved water sources: house connection, standpost, borehole, dug well, and rainwater collection.

Improving water supply can lead to a variety of health benefits. The most important studies that have been done have shown that providing a continuous supply of water with good bacteriological quality can reduce the morbidity of a number of diseases. Studies showed a median reduction in trachoma, for example, of 27%, schistosomiasis of 77%, and dracunculiasis of 78%.[10]

Other studies have looked at the health benefits from different combinations of investments in water quantity, water quality, sanitation, and the promotion of hygiene. The results of these studies are somewhat surprising to those not involved in the environmental health field. They suggest that the largest reductions in diarrhea morbidity—approximately 30%—come from investing in sanitation only, water and sanitation, or hygiene only. The lowest reductions, between 15 and 20%, came from investing in water quantity only, or a combination of water quality and quantity, all without complementary investments in hygiene or in sanitation.[10]

As noted earlier, many of the pathogens that are waterborne are also carried on food. Thus, sanitation has a large potential impact on reducing those pathogens. By contrast, investing in water interventions alone may not yield the results that sanitation would. For this, among other reasons, complementary investments for the promotion of hygiene are critical to realizing gains from water and sanitation.[10] Another important lesson is that the greatest effect of investments in water is realized when people have water connections in their homes. Unfortunately, community standpipes, for example, do not produce the same level of health gains as individual household water connections. Nonetheless, it is also important to realize that it is estimated that over 1 billion people engage in home treatment of water to improve its safety. In surveys of countries representing approximately

40% of the global population, about 36% of urban dwellers, and 30% of rural dwellers engaged in home water treatment, through boiling, filtration, chlorination, or solar disinfection.[21]

Hygiene

Unfortunately, there have been relatively few studies of the impact of hygiene promotion on actual health behaviors and on related reductions in the burden of disease. The studies that have been done showed that investing in hygiene promotion led to a 33% reduction in diarrhea. Studies have also been done on the impact of handwashing on respiratory infections. Handwashing was associated in these studies with a significant reduction in acute respiratory infections.[10]

Integrating Investment Choices About Water, Sanitation, and Hygiene

When the information from the studies previously discussed is reviewed together, it appears that the promotion of hygiene, the promotion of sanitation, and the construction of standposts are all likely to be cost-effective in low- and middle-income countries. The costs of hygiene and sanitation promotion compare favorably, for example, with the costs per DALY averted of oral rehydration. In addition, such investments might help to reduce the burden of diarrhea and decrease the need for oral rehydration.[10]

Climate Change and Health

Background

Climate change refers to the increase in the earth's average temperature that has been observed and the consequences that might be associated with this rise in temperature.[22] It is estimated that the earth has warmed by 1.5°F (0.8°C) in the past 100 years.[23] Accompanying the rising temperature has been a change in rainfall levels; an increase in the frequency of extreme weather, such as floods, droughts, and heat waves; and the melting of glaciers, warming of the oceans, and the rising of sea levels.[23] The United Nations Secretary-General has said that climate change is the major, overriding environmental issue of our time.[24] Climate change is also considered a significant threat to efforts to improve the health of poor people in the poorest countries.[25]

The Problem: A Range of Future Risks to Health

The United Nations Intergovernmental Panel on Climate Change (IPCC), the leading international body for the assessment of climate change, suggested that climate change thus far has had only a limited impact on human health. The panel further noted that the impacts on health to date have come largely through increased heat-related mortality and decreased cold-related mortality, plus temperature-related changes in the distribution of some waterborne and vector-borne diseases.[26]

The panel also noted, however, a range of future risks to health:

- Declines in the production of some food crops in some locations leading to increases in undernutrition in certain settings
- Increases in ill health in low-income countries due to more intense heat waves and fires, as well as increases in foodborne, waterborne, and vector-borne diseases

At the same time, there may be places that can increase food production and see a decline in these diseases. Nonetheless, the panel suggested that the negative impacts of climate change on health in this century will greatly outweigh the positive benefits.[26]

Considering these findings, WHO has estimated that climate change will cause an additional 250,000 deaths per year between 2030 and 2050. Specifically, WHO has estimated that climate change will lead to approximately 38,000 additional deaths annually due to heat exposure in elderly people, 48,000 deaths due to diarrhea, 60,000 deaths due to malaria, and 95,000 deaths due to childhood undernutrition.[25]

The IPCC concluded earlier that it is 95% certain that human activities have caused most of the warming of the planet's surface that has occurred since the 1950s. These findings place increased pressure on the global society to act to reverse the observed trends, especially because those predicted to be affected the most by the effects of climate change have contributed least to its causes.[23]

How Does Climate Change Affect Health?

There are many mechanisms through which climate change can affect health. For example, extreme weather patterns, such as droughts, flooding, and heat waves, can lead to direct increases in mortality as a result of their effect on infrastructure, disruption of daily activities, and severe conditions placed on the human body. Droughts are thought to have the greatest global disaster effects because they often affect large regions.[27] In addition, variable rainfall patterns can result in a lack of a safe water supply, which can compromise hygiene and can lead to increased risk of diarrheal disease.[27] Changes in rainfall can also indirectly affect the nutritional status of populations by altering agricultural production. Higher temperatures contribute to deaths associated with respiratory and cardiovascular disease as the body is subjected to harsher conditions. High temperatures can also exacerbate air pollution levels, which can lead to a greater incidence of asthma cases. Changing weather patterns can influence the balance of ecosystems and biodiversity of a region. Even small changes in rainfall and temperature can alter the distribution of disease carriers, such as mosquitoes, which can then affect the prevalence of vector-borne diseases, such as dengue or malaria.[28] It is anticipated that climate change will also be associated with substantial displacement of populations and a range of impacts on mental health.[29]

Who Is Affected?

All people are at risk of being negatively affected by climate change. Nonetheless, some groups of people are more vulnerable than others.[30] In particular, low-income countries, and in some cases middle-income countries as well, could be affected to a greater extent because areas with weak health infrastructure will be least prepared to respond and adapt to the changes in weather and corresponding changing health and disease patterns. The losses related to climate change are also much less likely to be insured in low-income countries than in other countries. One estimate, for example, suggested that 99% of climate-related losses in low-income countries since 1990 have not been covered by insurance.[29] In addition, it is anticipated that urban areas will be affected to a greater extent by any negative impacts of air pollution or rises in temperature, whereas rural areas will be more affected by changes in weather patterns that affect agricultural production.[25]

Within all countries, children and the elderly will be among the most vulnerable to the diseases climate change is likely to influence. Children will be affected by an increased risk of diarrheal disease, malaria, and undernutrition, whereas the elderly will be most affected by increased risk of heat-related conditions and extreme weather patterns, given their more fragile physical state.[25,31]

What Must Be Done?

Climate change is likely to have high human and economic costs. In fact, WHO estimates that by 2030, the damage to health will be between $2 billion and $4 billion per year.[25] The potential health and economic consequences can be mitigated with cost-effective interventions. The climate change response proposed by the United Nations Environment Programme involves both adaptation strategies that build resilience to climate change in the short run and mitigation strategies that aim to reduce long-term carbon emissions.[32] All mitigation and adaptation strategies offer direct health benefits as a result of either preventing the effects of climate change on health or preparing the health community to better respond to these effects.

In the short term, the public health community can prepare for any negative climate change effects by enhancing public health education surrounding emergency preparedness, warnings of high pollution, and general public health education, including boil water notices during floods, public awareness on vector-borne diseases, and promotion of good hygiene.[33]

In the long term, mitigation efforts revolve around reducing emissions of greenhouse gases, particularly carbon and methane emissions.[34] Assuming a world population of 9 billion by 2050, reductions of more than two-thirds in emissions would be needed to avoid doubling preindustrial revolution levels.[28] Effective control efforts would avoid 0.6 million to 4.4 million deaths related to particulate matter and 40,000 to 520,000 ozone-related deaths and can also increase annual crop yields by 30 million to 135 million metric tons due to ozone reductions in 2030 and beyond.[35,36] Benefits of methane emission reductions have been estimated at $700 to $5,000 per metric ton.[36]

The United Nations Environmental Programme suggests many strategies to control carbon and methane emissions, but given that the largest contributor to greenhouse emissions is the burning of fossil fuels, reducing this activity should be a priority.[36] Fossil fuels can be controlled both directly and indirectly. For example, on a policy level, regulations can be put in place that directly limit the magnitude of emissions or that require manufacturing processes that are more environmentally friendly and less wasteful.[34]

In addition, research and support of energy sources other than fossil fuels must be sustained as a mitigation strategy in order to offer an alternative to the burning of fossil fuels. These commitments need to be made in low- and middle-income countries, as well as in high-income countries, and there have already been successful and cost-effective interventions in resource-poor settings. In Jaipur, India, for example, a 350-bed health facility cut its total energy bill in half between 2005 and 2008 through solar-powered water heaters and lighting. In Brazil, one efficiency initiative reduced the demand for electricity of a group of 101 hospitals by 1,035 kilowatts at a cost savings of 25%.[31]

Another mitigation strategy is the halting of deforestation and forest degradation. Agricultural expansion, forest clearing, infrastructure development, destructive logging, fires, and other similar activities contribute almost 20% of global greenhouse gas emissions, the second-leading contributor.[37] These activities can be discouraged through offering alternative economic means for organizations and individuals engaged with them, such as creating carbon markets in which governments or businesses are rewarded for their efforts made to reduce carbon emissions.[34]

Other mitigation strategies can include reducing agricultural waste and inefficiency through investing in new farming and storing technologies, reducing waste associated with the construction industry, investing in improved recycling infrastructure, or promoting sustainable tourism that engages local communities and protects natural ecosystems.[34] A range of actors have stated that interventions must be implemented on the individual, local, national, and international levels in order to best mitigate the looming potential effects of climate change on health.[30]

Occupational Health

What Is Occupational Health?

Occupational health is a discipline that focuses on avoiding and reducing serious injuries and diseases among workers. However, occupational health also includes activities for improving the general well-being of workers in a workplace. There are several definitions of occupational health, but the one most commonly used is this definition from WHO and the International Labor Organization (ILO), first developed in 1950:

> Occupational health is: the promotion and maintenance of the highest degree of physical, mental, and social well-being of workers in all occupations.[37]

A more recent definition of **Occupational safety and health (OSH)** is:

> the science of the anticipation, recognition, evaluation and control of hazards arising in or from the workplace that could impair the health and well-being of workers, taking into account the possible impact on the surrounding communities and the general environment.[38]

Examples of Occupational Health Issues

Occupational health focuses on the prevention and reduction of unwanted health effects. It aims for safe and healthy workplaces and for keeping workers from becoming patients. Since many people are not very familiar with occupational health, some examples follow that illustrate key occupational health concepts:

- Work on building sites may cause serious accidents among workers, such as falling from scaffolding. This can be prevented by using strong scaffolding that is put up correctly, and by teaching the workers how to use the scaffolding safely. This type of preventive work may save the lives of many workers in the building industry.
- Patients with communicable diseases may transmit them to health workers, as has too often been the case for COVID-19. It is very important that health personnel have correct facemasks, gloves, and clothing, for example, to avoid being infected when treating patients.
- In East Africa, there are an increasing number of flower farms, especially farms growing roses. Roses are very popular in the high-income world, and large numbers of roses are exported from East Africa to Europe. These flower farms are huge and may employ thousands of people. However, the flower farms spray large amounts of pesticides on the roses every day to protect the plants. Most pesticides are very toxic and can cause serious poisoning among the workers. Providing information and appropriate equipment to workers to help them to use pesticides properly can prevent such poisoning.
- Miners work in a very dusty environment. The dust comes from drilling into rock. This type of dust can easily be inhaled and cause different types of lung diseases. An example is coal miners who may inhale large amounts of coal dust. They may develop a cough. After some time, the cough may worsen and serious breathing problems may develop. This is a typical start of the chronic and uncurable disease called "coal workers pneumoconiosis." Yet, this is a disease we can prevent through the use of personal protective equipment and by, for instance, using water during drilling to reduce the dust in the air.

Why Should We Care About the Health of Workers?

Workers represent about half of the world's population and are major contributors to socio-economic development.[39] Continued, sustainable socio-economic development is only possible if workers have a decent working environment. Sustainable Development Goal number 8 is "Promote sustained, inclusive and sustainable economic growth, full and productive employment and decent work for all."[40] Sub-goal 8.8 states: "Protect labor rights and promote safe and secure working environments for all workers by 2030."[41] Millions of men and women globally have poor and hazardous working conditions. Despite knowledge about effective interventions to prevent occupational hazards and to protect and promote health at the workplace, large gaps exist between and within countries regarding the health status of workers and their exposure to occupational risks. There needs to be increased awareness of dangerous workplaces and enhanced efforts to prevent occupational accidents and diseases.

The Burden of Disease Related to Occupational Health

The figures from different countries regarding employment and disease vary in quality and reliability, and calculation of the global burden of disease (GBD) related to occupational health is difficult to perform. Nonetheless, existing data suggest there is a very large burden of occupationally related illness, disability, and death.

ILO suggests that almost 2.8 million people a year die as a result of occupationally-related accidents or diseases.[42] This compares, for example, with 690,000 people who died of HIV/AIDS in 2019.[43] ILO also estimates that there are almost 375 million nonfatal work-related injuries in the world every year[44] and about 160 million people who suffer work-related illnesses each year.[44] ILO further suggests that hazardous substances alone cause more than 650,000 deaths a year, close to the number who die each year of HIV/AIDS.[44]

WHO reports that the occupational cancer burden is of major importance, exemplified by development of mesothelioma after asbestos exposure. In addition, cardiovascular diseases are an important part of the burden of disease related to occupational health, related, for instance, to noise, heat, chemical exposure, shift-work, and high psychological demands.[45]

ILO notes the disproportionately high number of reported accidents in the construction industry and disproportionate risks that both younger and older workers, including child workers, face.[44] Workers in low- and middle-income countries face higher risks of work-related injury or illness than workers in high-income countries. Workers in small enterprises face higher risks than those in large enterprises. Migrant workers tend to be employed in more dangerous work than others. Women appear to be at lower risk of workplace injuries than men, but this may relate largely to the different work they undertake in many settings. Agriculture, forestry, fishing, manufacturing, construction, and transportation are the riskiest sectors within which to work. Earlier studies suggest that about 80% of all occupationally-related deaths in the world each year occur in low- and middle-income countries. The lack of health and safety regulations or weak capacity to implement them are also important risk factors for occupationally-related injuries and illnesses.[46]

The Economic Consequences of Occupational Health Issues

The inadequate prevention of occupational diseases has profound negative effects not only on workers and their families but also on society at large due to the tremendous associated costs, particularly in terms of loss of productivity and the burden to social security systems. The European Agency for Safety and Health at Work (EU-OSHA) has estimated that 3.9% of global gross national product (GNP) and 3.3% of European GNP is spent on occupational injuries and diseases. Similarly, ILO estimates the overall economic loss from work-related diseases and injuries to be 4% of the world's GNP. The percentage may vary widely between countries, in particular between low-, middle-, and high-income countries, depending on the industrial mix, legislative context, and prevention incentives.[47]

Critical Constraints to Enhancing Occupational Health

Occupational health services aim to lower risk factors at work, implement health surveillance and training in safe working methods, provide first aid, and act as consultants for employers on health and safety. Even though this benefits the workers, access to occupational health services is not available in many countries. This is despite the United Nations position that the absence of occupational health services is a violation of the right to health.[48]

Why is this the case? Globally, much is known about occupational health. However, its implementation in health systems and at workplaces is lacking in many countries, probably due to lack of competence and political will. The expanding labor market and rapid changes in work situations in many countries creates highly competitive industrial settings globally. Expenses related to occupational health services are not prioritized. The situation is often worsened by governments who prioritize the establishment of new industrial activities in their countries but focus less on care for the workers. In addition, labor unions are weak in many countries and not strong enough to influence politicians and stakeholders.

Most countries have a specific law, "A Working Environment Act," to ensure that working environments do not harm employees. However, different countries interpret and implement such laws in different ways. Many countries have a labor inspectorate that performs controls. However, many labor inspectorates have few resources. In addition, labor inspectors often lack the authority to enforce penalties on industries that do not follow the existing rules.

Addressing Key Occupational Health Issues

There are a number of measures that need to be taken to enhance occupational health and safety, particularly in low- and middle-income countries. These must vary by country and could include, as appropriate to the setting, some of the following:[47]

- Primary prevention—such as personal protective equipment
- Enhancing healthcare and rehabilitative services related to occupational injuries
- Developing a competent occupational health workforce
- Improving the data on occupational injuries
- Strengthening regulations and enforcement of matters related to occupational injury
- Training workers and managers in recognizing and controlling hazards, implementing safe work practices to reduce risk, dissemination of safety and health information, and strengthening emergency procedures
- Taking participatory approaches to enhancing ergonomics of working environments
- Measures to prevent falls from heights
- Taking a systemic approach to dealing with psychosocial risks

Intersectoral Approaches to Enabling Better Health[49]

Key Definition

Most global health issues are intersectoral in nature. This section focuses briefly on the importance of taking a broad view of health and on the role of "intersectoral approaches" to improving health. Such approaches can be defined in the following way:

> Actions undertaken by sectors outside the health sector, possibly, but not necessarily, in collaboration with the health sector, on health or health equity outcomes or on the determinants of health or health equity.[50]

The Role of Intersectoral Approaches in Addressing the Determinants of Health and Health Risk Factors

With the above in mind, let's ask ourselves the following:

- What is the extent to which the determinants of health and critical risk factors can be addressed by actions within the health sector?
- What is the extent to which they can be addressed only through actions by agencies outside of the health sector or by those agencies in collaboration with the health sector?

A few examples highlight the importance of addressing health issues in intersectoral ways. Several key risk factors for diabetes, for example, relate to nutrition. These can be most comprehensively addressed with support from outside of the health sector. Appropriate infant and child feeding practices depend on the level of education of the caregivers and their ability to buy healthy foods for their children. These relate largely to policies on education, agriculture, and a range of social matters. In addition, a person's health depends on access to safe water and sanitation, which relates mostly to infrastructure policies and programs. A person's ability to get enough physical activity depends partly on access to recreational facilities and the extent to which people see them as safe. These generally fall under the purview of urban planners and law enforcement agencies. Agencies outside of the health sector are also central to controlling tobacco and ambient particulate matter pollution.

Policy and Program Approaches to Addressing Intersectoral Issues

The "Whole of Government" or "Health in All Policies" Approach

There are several ways in which countries can organize themselves to address health issues that require an intersectoral approach.[51] One approach is called "health in all policies" or a "whole of government" approach. In this case, all ministries in a government are required to account for the health implications of their policies, plans, and programs. To varying degrees, Cuba, England, New Zealand, and Norway take such an approach to improving the health of their populations. The central government of these countries asks *all* government agencies to work together to maximize the health of their people and/or to reduce inequities in health.[52]

Achieving a successful "health in all policies" approach, however, may require more organizational and management capacity than may be available in some low- and middle-income countries.[51] Nonetheless, most of these countries could seek opportunities to work across sectors on specific health issues that require an intersectoral approach. The government, for example, might choose to address some of the biggest risks, such as tobacco, with an intersectoral approach. A coordinating committee could then oversee that effort.[52] The ministry of health could engage in health awareness activities about tobacco; the ministry of commerce could limit advertising, sales to minors, and sales hours; the ministry of agriculture could promote alternative crops for tobacco farmers; and the ministry of finance could oversee the raising of taxes on tobacco.

Health Impact Assessments

Governments also might gain a better understanding of the intersectoral actions needed to address some health issues by carrying out a **health impact assessment**.[53] A health impact assessment has been defined by WHO as follows:

> A combination of procedures, methods and tools by which a policy, program or project may be judged as to its potential effects on the health of a population, and the distribution of those effects within the population.[53]

The purpose of the health impact assessment is to examine the health consequences of activities across a range of economic sectors. The findings of health impact assessments should provide policymakers with the information they need to maximize the positive effects of investments and minimize the negative effects.

The most effective health impact assessments do the following:[54]

- Bring together and take account of the views of a wide range of stakeholders
- Take a broad perspective by looking at social, economic, and environmental issues, among other factors
- Examine *whose* health is likely to be affected by the investment that is being assessed
- Provide policymakers with data-driven recommendations about how to minimize the adverse effects of the proposed investment and maximize its health gains

Let's examine briefly why health impact assessments can be so valuable. Investments in roads, for example, might produce substantial economic benefits. At the same time, the construction of the road and the road itself might be associated with pooling water and an increase in mosquito-borne diseases or an increase in traffic injuries. The use of fertilizer and pesticides can produce larger crop yields, which can help address undernutrition and improve young child health. However, if not used properly, these chemicals might lead to poisonings among some of the people who handle them. New manufacturing plants can create job opportunities and other economic benefits, but if not regulated carefully, they might also lead to increased air pollution or toxic industrial waste. If health impact assessments are carried out during the planning of investments like those noted above, governments can identify potential health risks of the investment and propose measures for preventing or mitigating them.

Putting Together an Intersectoral Policy Package

A recent study examined the importance of intersectoral approaches to addressing environmental, social, and behavioral risk factors and how they might be structured in different country settings. That study concluded that intersectoral policies could usefully be divided into four categories: taxes and subsidies, regulation and related enforcement mechanisms, policies related to the built environment, and policies concerning the provision of information. The study identified 79 intersectoral policies to be of greatest priority. The study further concluded that about half of those policies should be adopted at an early stage, even in low-income and lower middle-income countries.[49]

The study also highlighted that those countries that have been able to make the most progress in reducing air pollution and road traffic injuries took an intersectoral approach.[48] The study also focuses attention on the exceptional importance of the ministry of finance in helping to lead and to address health risks. That ministry, for example, would deal with taxes on tobacco and alcohol. That ministry also might levy taxes on sugar or sugary beverages or on highly polluting processes, such as vehicular emissions. In addition, the ministry of finance could limit subsidies that are detrimental to health, such as those encouraging the production of unhealthy food or fossil fuels.[49]

Discussion Questions

1. Why do low-income people suffer disproportionately from environmental health risks?
2. Why is household air pollution such an important risk factor in low-income settings? What are the most cost-efficient ways to reduce such risks?
3. Why does investing in water quantity alone fail to yield the benefits that come from investing in water quantity and better hygiene at the same time?
4. How large is the burden of deaths related to occupationally related injuries and diseases compared with other major causes of deaths? Why is this burden so large?
5. Why is it so important to take an all-in-government approach to dealing with some of the most important causes of death and disability?

References

1. Cohen AJ, Brauer M, Burnett R, et al. Estimates and 25-year trends of the global burden of disease attributable to ambient air pollution: an analysis of data from the Global Burden of Diseases Study 2015. *Lancet.* 2017;389(10082):1907–1918.

2. McMichael AJ, Kjellstrom T, Smith KR. Environmental health. In: Merson MH, Black RE, Mills A, eds. *International Public Health: Diseases, Programs, Systems, and Policies.* Gaithersburg, MD: Aspen; 2001.

3. The World Bank. *Environmental health at a glance.* nd. Washington, DC. © World Bank. Retrieved from https://openknowledge.worldbank.org/handle/10986/9734 License:CC BY 3.0 IGO

4. McMillan A, Kjellstrom T, Smith KR, Pillarisetti A, Woodward A. Environmental and occupational health. Merson M, Mills A, Black R, eds. In: Merson M, Black R, Mills A, eds. *Global Health Disease Systems, Programs, and Policies.* 4th ed. Burlington, MA: 2018: 479.

5. World Health Organization. *Household air pollution and health: key facts.* 2018. Retrieved from http://www.who.int/en/news-room/fact-sheets/detail/household-air-pollution-and-health

6. Yassi A, Kjellstrom T, de Kok T, Guidotti TL. Air. In: *Basic Environmental Health.* New York, NY: Oxford University Press; 2001:180–208.

7. Yassi A, Kjellstrom T, de Kok T, Guidotti TL. Health and energy use. In: *Basic Environmental Health.* New York, NY: Oxford University Press;2001:311–331.

8. World Health Organization. *Drinking-water.* 2019. Retrieved from https://www.who.int/news-room/fact-sheets/detail/drinking-water

9. World Health Organization. *Sanitation.* 2019. Retrieved from https://www.who.int/news-room/fact-sheets/detail/sanitation

10. Cairncross S, Valdmanis V. Water supply, sanitation, and hygiene promotion. In: Jamison DT, Breman JG, Measham AR, et al., eds. *Disease Control Priorities in Developing Countries.* 2nd ed. New York, NY: Oxford University Press; 2006: 771–792.

11. UNICEF. *Hygiene.* 2021. Retrieved from https://data.unicef.org/topic/water-and-sanitation/hygiene/

12. Institute of Health Metrics and Evaluation. *GBD Compare|Viz Hub.* nd. Retrieved from: https://vizhub.healthdata.org/gbd-compare/

13. World Health Organization.*Ambient (outdoor) air pollution.* 2018. Retrieved from https://www.who.int/news-room/fact-sheets/detail/ambient-(outdoor)-air-quality-and-health

14. Landrigan PJ, Fuller R, Acosta NJR, et al. The Lancet Commission on pollution and health. *The Lancet.* 2018;391(10119):462–512.

15. Feachem R, Bradley D, Garelick H, Mara D. *Sanitation and Disease: Health Aspects of Excreta and Wastewater Management.* Chichester, UK: John Wiley & Sons; 1983.

16. Prüss-Ustün A, Bartram J, Clasen T, et al. Burden of disease from inadequate water, sanitation and hygiene in low- and middle-income settings: a retrospective analysis of data from 145 countries. *Trop Med Int Health.* 2014;19(8):894–905.

17. Kjellstrom T, Lodh M, McMichael AJ, Ranmuthugala G, Shrestha R, Kingsland S. Air and water pollution: burden and strategies for control. In: Jamison DT, Breman G, Measham AR, et al., eds. *Disease Control Priorities in Developing Countries.* 2nd ed. New York, NY: Oxford University Press; 2006:817–832.

18. Bruce N, Rehfuess E, Mehta S, Hutton G, Smith K. Household air pollution. In: Jamison DT, Breman JG, Measham AR, et al., eds. *Disease Control Priorities in Developing Countries.* 2nd ed. New York, NY: Oxford University Press; 2006: 793–816.

19. Allan S. *The WaterAid Bangladesh/VERC 100% Sanitation Approach: Cost, Motivation and Subsidy.* Unpublished Master's thesis, London School of Hygiene; 2003.

20. Emerson PM, Lindsay SW, Alexander N, et al. Role of flies and provision of latrines in trachoma control: cluster-randomised controlled trial. *Lancet.* 2004;363(9415):1093–1098.

21. Rosa G, Thomas, C. Estimating the scope of household water treatment in low- and medium-income countries. *Am J Trop Med Hyg.* 2010;82(2):289–300.

22. Environmental Protection Agency. *Climate change: basic information.* 2017. Retrieved from https://19january2017snapshot.epa.gov/climatechange/climate-change-basic-information_.html

23. Intergovernmental Panel on Climate Change. *Climate change 2014: impacts, adaptation, and vulnerability. Summary for policymakers.* UK: Cambridge University Press; 2014:6.
24. United Nations Secretary-General. (2017). *Secretary-General on climate action (as delivered).* Retrieved from https://www.un.org/sg/en/content/sg/statement/2017-05-30/secretary-general -climate-action-delivered
25. World Health Organization. *Climate change and health: key facts.* 2018. Retrieved from http://www.who.int/news-room/fact-sheets/detail/climate-change-and-health
26. Intergovernmental Panel on Climate Change. *Climate change 2013: the physical science basis.* Contribution of Working Group I to the fifth assessment report of the Intergovernmental Panel on Climate Change. Cambridge, UK: Cambridge University Press; 2013.
27. McMichael AJ, Woodruff RE, Hales S. Climate change and human health: present and future risks. *Lancet.* 2006;367(9513):859–869.
28. Haines A, Kovats RS, Campbell-Lendrum D, Corvalan C. Climate change and human health: impacts, vulnerability and public health. *Public Health.* 2006;120(7):585–596.
29. Watts N, Amann M, Ayeb-Karlsson S, et al. The Lancet countdown on health and climate change: From 25 years of inaction to a global transformation for public health. *Lancet.* 2018;391(10120):581–630.
30. Costello A, Abbas M, Allen A, et al. Managing the health effects of climate change. *Lancet.* 2009;37(9676):1693–1733. doi: 10.1016/S0140-6736(09)60935-1
31. Neira M. *Environmental health and sustainable development.* Geneva, Switzerland: World Health Organization. 2012. Retrieved from http://ec.europa.eu/environment/archives/soil /pdf/may2012/02%20-%20Maria%20Neira%20-% 20final.pdf
32. United Nations Environment Programme. *Climate change.* nd. Retrieved from https://www .unenvironment.org/explore-topics/climate-change
33. United Nations Environment Programme. *Climate change adaptation.* nd. Retrieved from https://www.unenvironment.org/explore-topics/climate-change/what-we-do/climate -adaptation
34. United Nations Environment Programme. *Climate change mitigation.* nd. Retrieved from https:// www.unenvironment.org/explore-topics/climate-change/what-we-do/mitigation
35. Anenberg SC, Schwartz J, Shindell D, et al. Global air quality and health co-benefits of mitigating near-term climate change through methane and black carbon emission controls. *Environ Health Perspect.* 2012;120(6):831–839.
36. Shindell D, Kuylenstierna JC, Vignati A, et al. Simultaneously mitigating near-term climate change and improving human health and food security. *Science.* 2012;335(6065):183–189.
37. HE&W. What is occupational health? nd. Retrieved from http://www.agius.com/hew/resource /ohsilo.htm
38. Alli, BO. *Fundamental principles of occupational health and safety.* Geneva, Switzerland: International Labor Organization; 2008.
39. World Bank. Data. *Labor force, total.* nd. Retrieved from https://data.worldbank.org/indicator /SL.TLF.TOTL.IN
40. United Nations. *The 17 goals.* nd. Retrieved from https://sdgs.un.org/goals
41. United Nations. *Goals 8.* nd. Retrieved from: https://sdgs.un.org/goals/goal8
42. International Labor Organization. *Safety and health at work.* nd. Retrieved from https://www .ilo.org/global/topics/safety-and-health-at-work/lang--en/index.htm
43. UNAIDS. *Global HIV & AIDS statistics – 2020 fact sheet.* nd. Retrieved from https://www.unaids .org/en/resources/fact-sheet
44. International Labor Organization. *World statistic.* nd. Retrieved from https://www.ilo.org /moscow/areas-of-work/occupational-safety-and-health/WCMS_249278/lang--en/index.htm
45. Koh D, Aw T-C. Textbook of occupational medicine practice. 4th ed. World Scientific Publishing Co., 2018:403–436.
46. Abdalla S, Apramian SS, Cantley LF, Cullen MR. Occupation and risk for injuries. In: Mock CN, Nugent R, Kobusingye O, et al., eds. *Disease Control Priorities.* 3rd ed. The International Bank for Reconstruction and Development/The World Bank; Washington, DC. 2017:6.
47. Takala J, Hämäläinen P, Saarela KL, et al. Global estimates of the burden of injury and illness at work in 2021. *J Occ Environ Hyg.* 2014;11:326–337.

48. United Nations General Assembly of Human Rights Council. Report of the Special Rapporteur on the right of everyone to the enjoyment of the highest attainable standard of physical and mental health, Anand Grover. 2012.

49. Watkins DA, Nugent R, Saxenian H, et al. Intersectoral policy priorities for health. In: Jamison DT, Gelband H, Horton S, et al., eds. *Disease Control Priorities: Improving Health and Reducing Poverty.* 3rd ed. Washington, DC: The World Bank; 2018: 23–42.

50. Public Health Agency of Canada and World Health Organization. *Health Equity Through Intersectoral Action: An Analysis of 18 Country Case Studies.* 2008. Retrieved from http://www .who.int/social_determinants/resources/health_equity_isa_2008_en.pdf

51. Khayatzadeh-Mahani A, Sedoghi Z, Mehrolhassani MH, Yazdi-Feyzabadi V. How health in all policies are developed and implemented in a developing country? A case study of a HiAP initiative in Iran. *Health Promotion International.* 2016;31(4):769–781. doi: 10.1093/heapro /dav062

52. World Health Organization. *Intersectoral action on health: A path for policy-makers to implement effective and sustainable action on health.* 2011. Retrieved from http://www.who.int/kobe _centre/publications/intersectorial_action_health2011/en/

53. World Health Organization. *Health impact assessment (HIA): Definitions of HIA.* nd. Retrieved from http://www.who.int/hia/about/defin/en/

54. The Pew Charitable Trusts. *Health Impact Project: Health impact assessment.* nd. Retrieved from http://www.pewtrusts.org/en/projects/health-impact-project/health-impact-assessment

CHAPTER 5

Nutrition and the Health of Women, Children, Adolescents, and Young Adults

Courtesy of Mark Tuschman

LEARNING OBJECTIVES

By the end of this chapter, the reader will be able to do the following:

- Discuss the importance of nutrition to health, the key issues of undernutrition and obesity and overweight, and critical measures to address these issues
- Review the leading causes of deaths and disability-adjusted life years (DALYs) in females worldwide and evidence-based measures to reduce premature deaths and disability among females
- Highlight the leading causes of death among children under five years of age and what measures can be taken to reduce such deaths
- Note the leading causes of deaths and DALYs among adolescents and young adults and evidence-based measures to reduce death and disability in these groups

VIGNETTES

Rachel and her mother lived in Mombasa, Kenya. Rachel had already received her first polio vaccine, and she would soon get another. When the children participated in "polio days," they not only got a polio vaccine but also a dose of vitamin A. There used to be many young children in Kenya and elsewhere who were blind due to the lack of vitamin A. Almost no children had become blind, however, since the vitamin A program had begun.

Sarah lived in rural Pakistan and was pregnant with her second child. When she went into labor, Sarah called for the traditional birth attendant, as most women did in her town. As Sarah's labor continued, she and the birth attendant realized that the labor was complicated. Sarah needed to go to a hospital to deliver the baby. In this part of Pakistan, however, women could not be taken to hospitals without their husband's permission. Sarah's husband was working in another city and was not available to give such permission. Several hours later, Sarah and the baby died at Sarah's home.

Juan was born in the highlands of Bolivia to an indigenous family. The family did what they could to keep the new baby warm, but it was very cold in the mountains. Several days after birth, Juan began to breathe heavily. The family called the community health worker for assistance. The health worker treated Juan for pneumonia with an antibiotic for saving newborn lives that she had just learned to use through a community-based program. She also gave the family advice about taking care of the baby. The last child born to the family had died of pneumonia, but Juan survived.

Rashmi is a 14-year-old girl in the Punjab state in India. She is hardworking and very intelligent but always feels great pressure to meet the expectations of her family and community. She worries all of the time about how she can complete her chores at home, help earn money for the family, do well in school, and then marry the young man her family will choose for her. Lately, her body has gone through a number of changes that she does not understand, and she has begun to feel more and more sad about all that she has to do. She feels like something is wrong but does not know what it is or what to do about it.

Introduction to the Chapter

This chapter covers a range of related topics as it reviews nutrition, as well as the health of women, young children, adolescents, and young adults. Given the breadth of the chapter, it can only be introductory. Each of the chapter topics is worthy of considerable additional study, which those reading this book are encouraged to do.

Nutrition

The Importance of Nutrition

Nutritional status is a major determinant of health status. It has an important bearing on the health of pregnant women and on pregnancy outcomes for both mothers and children. It is a major determinant of the birthweight of children, how children grow, and the extent to which their cognitive functions develop properly. Nutritional status is also closely linked with the strength of one's immune system and one's ability to stay healthy. In fact, approximately 45% of young child deaths in low- and middle-income countries have been attributed to causes related to **undernutrition**.[1] At the same time, however, childhood **obesity** has become an enormous challenge, in part because it tends to continue into adulthood, increasing the risk of chronic diseases later in life.[2]

In addition, nutritional status has an important bearing on people's capacity to learn and on their productivity. Nutritional deficits can seriously hamper the ability of children to attend school, concentrate while they are there, and learn effectively. Numerous studies have shown that workers who are anemic produce less than workers who do not suffer from **iron deficiency anemia**. Obesity and **overweight** also affect worker productivity.[3]

The Nutritional State of the World

The nutritional picture of the world has changed dramatically in the last several decades, from one in which there was a preponderance of undernutrition to one in which there are now more people who suffer more from overweight and obesity than undernourishment. In addition, the vast majority of people who suffer from **malnutrition** live in low- and middle-income countries. Many countries will have to deal simultaneously for some time to come with a range of nutrition issues, including **underweight** and **micronutrient deficiencies**, as well as overweight and obesity.

When considering the nutritional state of the world, we must take account of **food security**, **low birthweight**, underweight, **stunting**, **wasting**, and overweight and obesity. WHO estimates that about 144 million children in the world who are under five years of age are stunted, 47 million are wasted, and more than 14 million are **severely wasted**. It is also estimated that more than 400 million adults are underweight. At the same time, about 1.9 billion adults are thought to have overweight or obesity.[4]

The share of low birthweight babies varied by country income group from 7.3% in upper middle-income countries to 19.9% in lower middle-income countries in 2015.[5] The regions with the highest share of low birthweight babies were Latin America and the Caribbean (9%) and East Asia and the Pacific (8%).[6] The same patterns are true for stunting: high-income countries will have almost no stunted children; however, low-income countries and even some middle-income countries, such as Guatemala, have rates above 40%.[7] Wasting varied in 2019 from being almost nonexistent in high-income countries to 6.6% in low-income countries; sub-Saharan Africa (6.8%) and South Asia (14.8%) have the highest rates of wasting.[8]

From the global health perspective, the most important concerns related to undernutrition are breastfeeding practices, whether people get enough of the right foods to have sufficient energy and protein, and the extent to which people have a sufficient intake of vitamin A, iodine, iron, zinc, and calcium. The importance of these nutrients and micronutrients varies with the place of people in their life course, with needs differing for infants, children, adolescents, pregnant and lactating women, adults, and older adults.

The prevalence of overweight and obesity has been increasing over the past decades. Globally, over 39% of adults and 18% of children and adolescents have overweight or have obesity.[9] The prevalence of obesity in WHO regions varies from 4.7% in South-East Asia to 28.6% in the Americas.[10] Obesity rates also vary by sex, with women generally having higher rates than men, varying from 6.1% in South-East Asia to 31% in the Americas.[10]

Micronutrient deficiencies are also critical and extensive. Although data on micronutrients are not updated as much as other nutrition data, there are high rates of iron deficiency anemia, iodine deficiency, and deficiency in vitamin A in selected regions, with low and middle-income countries being disproportionately impacted.[11] In 2016, 60% of children under five in sub-Saharan Africa and 50% of women of reproductive age (15–49) in South Asia[12] were anemic.[13] A recent study suggests that half of all children in the countries for which there were data showed zinc deficiency.[14]

The Determinants of Nutritional Status

Nutritional status is determined by a range of related and intersectoral issues. These can be divided into three levels:

- *Basic Causes at the Societal Level:* Such as resources available at the local level and the local environment and how they are organized and controlled.
- *Underlying Causes at the Household and Family Level:* Such as access to food, maternal and childcare, and access to water, sanitation, and health care.
- *Immediate Causes:* Such as disease and inadequate dietary intake.

Clearly, nutritional status relates in important ways to whether or not people have the income to purchase enough food or food of appropriate quality. However, nutritional status also relates to culture, customs, and eating behaviors. It is linked to agricultural markets, climate, and civil conflict as well. Malnutrition of all types disproportionately affects poor people, marginalized people, and females.

The growth of obesity and overweight has been driven by the interplay of genetic, behavioral, and environmental factors. Macrolevel forces, including global financial and trade liberalization, increased income and socioeconomic status, and urbanization have driven societal change, including changes to the food environment, the built environment, and socioeconomic and cultural influences. These changes, in turn, affect individual behaviors, diet, and physical activity. Genetic factors underlying susceptibility to weight gain may be amplified in the presence of certain environmental factors. The interaction of all of these factors has resulted in increased weight gain worldwide.[15]

The Effects of Malnutrition

Energy and protein malnutrition is associated with low birthweight, being underweight, failing to grow properly, and a weakening of immunity.[16] Vitamin A deficiency is well known for its impact on vision but is also closely associated with general immunity and child growth.[17] The lack of iron is the primary cause of iron deficiency anemia, which leads to weakness and fatigue; however, it is also associated with maternal morbidity and mortality, poor and stunted growth in children, and poor mental development in children.[18] The lack of iodine causes thyroid problems, goiter, and important deficits in mental abilities. Iodine is also essential for proper child growth.[18] Zinc is associated with general immunity, the growth of children, and the development of children's cognitive and motor abilities.[18]

About 45% of the deaths in the world today of children under five years of age are associated with undernutrition. The largest share of these deaths relates to stunting and underweight. The next largest relates to the joint effects of fetal growth restriction and suboptimal breastfeeding. More than 10% are attributable to wasting.[1,14]

Obesity and overweight are major risk factors for morbidity and mortality for a range of noncommunicable diseases, including cardiovascular disease, type 2 diabetes, hypertension, musculoskeletal disorders, and some forms of cancer.[19]

In 2017, high BMI contributed to 8.5% of deaths (4.7 million) and 5.8% of DALYs (147.7 million) globally. Obesity and overweight are now responsible, in fact, for more deaths than those attributable to undernutrition.[20]

Addressing Nutrition Challenges

Undernutrition

There are cost-effective solutions to undernutrition, as noted below. It is also critical to remember that the window of opportunity for ensuring that children are well nourished and develop properly is a small one. It begins at conception and lasts until children are about 2 years of age. Damage done to children's development in this period is largely irreversible.[21]

The most critical interventions to deal with undernutrition, which should be focused on South Asia and sub-Saharan Africa and on poor and marginalized communities elsewhere, are as follows: ensure that pregnant women are well nourished and have sufficient micronutrients; promote exclusive breastfeeding until six months of age; encourage the provision of appropriate complementary foods beginning at six months of age; support effective programs in supplementation and fortification, based on nutritional needs at the local level, and embed them in community-based approaches; fight infection and illness through improved water, sanitation, and hygiene; immunization; and better health and eating behaviors.[22-25]

Overweight and Obesity

The worldwide increase in overweight, obesity, and related chronic diseases has largely been driven by globalization, through a combination of global trade liberalization, economic growth, and rapid urbanization. These factors are causing dramatic changes in diet, lifestyles, and living environments, in turn promoting positive energy balance through interactions with genetic factors that make some people more susceptible to weight gain. Nutritional transitions in low- and middle-income countries involve increased consumption of fast food, increased prevalence of supermarkets, and a diet heavy in added sugar and animal products. Coupled with reductions in physical activity, and linked behavioral, cultural, and biological factors, obesity and overweight are increasing at alarming rates, especially in low- and middle-income countries.

Macrolevel changes are ultimately needed to prevent obesity, as they affect individual diet and physical activity. A diet with an emphasis on vegetables, fruits, whole grains, plant oils, and healthful sources of protein, such as fish, poultry, nuts, seeds, and beans, is crucial for health promotion. Health-promoting diets also include limited amounts of red and processed meats, saturated and trans fats, added sugars, salt, and refined carbohydrates. Reasonable portion sizes are also key for health, as is regular physical activity.[26]

Unfortunately, the vast majority of the world is not consuming a health-promoting diet or getting enough physical activity, as reflected by the 2.3 billion people worldwide who have overweight or obesity. In high-income countries, poorer people are most at risk for obesity and overweight, whereas in low- and middle-income countries, the wealthier are at a higher risk. Childhood obesity is of particular concern, as 38 million children under five had overweight or obesity as of 2016 and will likely continue this trend into adulthood.[27]

Prevention strategies across multiple levels are paramount, particularly in low- and middle-income countries that must manage a double burden of malnutrition. Changes should include high-level global policies from the international community to identify nutritional goals and guidelines. In addition, coordinated efforts by governments, organizations, communities, and individuals will be required to positively influence behavioral and environmental change. Policies and prevention efforts must also involve industry, the media, doctors, farmers, and urban planners.

Some of the most important and cost-effective interventions for addressing overweight, obesity, and the dietary risks to good health include measures that can be taken by governments, by industry, and by individuals:

- *Reduce sodium intake:* Through industry reformulation of packaged and restaurant foods, government-mandated labeling, expanding lower-sodium offerings in public institutions, and implementing mass-media behavior change campaigns.[28]
- *Reduce added sugar:* Through taxation, advertising restrictions, government-mandated labeling, and restricted offerings in public institutions.[29]
- *Eliminate Trans Fats:* Through a government-mandated ban, replace trans fats and saturated fats with unsaturated fats through reformulation, labeling, fiscal policies, or agricultural policies.[30]
- *Educate consumers:* Through mass media on diet and physical activity.[31]
- *Provide Preventive Care:* Through counseling and drug therapy for people with a high risk of developing heart attacks and strokes and through preventive foot care, retinopathy screening, and effective glycemic control for people with diabetes.[32]

As countries confront undernutrition, overweight, and obesity, it is essential to highlight the fact that addressing nutrition problems of all types will require action in three domains: nutrition-specific, nutrition-sensitive, and areas related to the enabling environment for nutrition.[22]

The Health of Females

Being Born Female Is Dangerous to Your Health

A well-known scholar and practitioner of women's health noted that "being born female is dangerous for your health."[33] Some of the health conditions that females face are biologically determined. Others are socially determined. Some result from the interplay between biological and social determinants of health. The inferior social status of females in many cultures, however, is reflected in certain health conditions that females face and in some of the differentials that favor men when considering the health of males and females.

The Burden of Disease for Females 15–49

It is important to think broadly of the health of females and go beyond the traditional focus on reproductive health issues. In low-income countries, the three leading causes of deaths of females aged 15–49 are HIV/AIDS, maternal disorders, and tuberculosis (TB), which are all Group I causes,[34] but stroke is the fourth leading cause and ischemic heart disease is the 10th leading cause. The same Group I causes are of special importance for females of this age group in lower middle-income countries, but ischemic heart disease and breast cancer rise in importance in this group.[34] As one moves to upper middle-income countries, HIV/AIDS continues to be important, but road injuries, ischemic heart disease, stroke, and breast cancer are also in the top five causes of death.[34] In high-income countries, breast cancer is the leading cause of death in this age group; self-harm, drug-use disorders, road injuries, and ischemic heart disease are also in the top five causes of death.[34]

The picture changes somewhat when we look at DALYs. For low-income countries, the five leading causes of DALYs among females in this age group are HIV/AIDS, maternal disorders, gynecological diseases, TB, and depressive disorders. In high-income countries, the five leading causes are low back pain, headache disorders, gynecological diseases, depressive disorders, and drug-use disorders.[34]

The main point to take away from these data is that Group I causes remain very important among poorer females, especially in poorer countries. However, ischemic heart disease, stroke, self-harm, road injuries, and a range of noncommunicable diseases are also among the leading causes of death among females, and they are rising in relative importance in this group.

Additional Comments on Selected Health Problems of Importance Among Females

Maternal Causes

About 295,000 women died in 2017 of maternal causes. The most immediate causes of maternal death are complications related to severe bleeding, generally after birth; post-birth infections; conditions related to high blood pressure; complications from delivery; and unsafe abortion. However, some of the more underlying causes of maternal death include anemia in the mother, stunting in the mother, young age at marriage and young age at first birth, having more than five children, and having closely spaced pregnancies. The lack of access to family planning is also at the foundation of some of these problems. In addition, women die maternal deaths when they cannot get access to timely emergency obstetric care of appropriate quality. It is essential to understand that the lifetime risk of a maternal death is only one in 5,400 in high-income countries but is one in 45 in low-income countries.[35]

It is also important to note the large number of women who suffer morbidity, often permanent, from the complications of pregnancy. Between 50,000 to 100,000 women each year, for example, are thought to suffer an **obstetric fistula** as a result of **obstructed labor**.[36]

Unsafe Abortion

The latest estimates suggest that about 29% of all pregnancies end with an **induced abortion**.[37] Each year, there are about 39 induced abortions for every 1,000 women of reproductive age, with the highest rates in low- and middle-income countries.[38] It is thought that about 55% of all abortions are **safe**. However, around 45% are unsafe. Almost all of the unsafe abortions occur in low- and middle-income countries. About 7 million women a year are admitted to hospitals as a result of unsafe abortion, and it has been estimated that between 5 and 13% of all maternal deaths can be attributed to unsafe abortions.[38]

Female Genital Mutilation

Female genital mutilation (FGM) is sometimes called **female genital cutting (FGC)** or is referred to as female genital mutilation/cutting.[39] WHO has recently estimated that almost 200 million females worldwide have been cut, predominantly in 30 countries in which FGM is concentrated. These countries are generally in west, east, or northeastern Africa and selected countries in the Middle East and Asia. It was estimated until recently that half of the girls who undergo FGM will be cut before they are five years of age and the remainder will be cut before they are 15 years of age. The cutting is generally done with razor blades, knives, or glass.[40] Female genital mutilation is very closely related to ethnicity. In addition, the higher the level of education of the mother, the less likely the daughter is to be cut.[41] The practice of FGM appears to be diminishing in Africa but staying around the same level in Asia.[41]

When FGM is performed initially, it can result in terrible pain or shock. It is also associated with infection. Over the longer term, it can lead to the retention of urine, infertility, and obstructed labor. Those more severely cut are more likely than others to have postpartum hemorrhage, caesarean section, and long stays in the hospital. In addition, the babies of such women are more likely than babies born to mothers who have not undergone FGM to need resuscitation immediately after birth, to be stillborn, or to die a neonatal death. If infection and hemorrhage linked to the act of FGM are not addressed in a timely and appropriate manner, FGM can also lead to death.[41]

Sexually Transmitted Infections Other than HIV/AIDS

Women are more biologically susceptible to sexually transmitted infections and their impact because they have more exposed mucosal surfaces, because they often show no symptoms of those diseases, and because their roles in society make them less likely to get treated for sexually transmitted infections than men.[42]

WHO estimates that each year there are over 350 million new infections with one of four STIs: chlamydia, gonorrhea, syphilis, and trichomoniasis. WHO further estimates that more than 500 million people worldwide have an infection with herpes simplex virus (HSV) and that more than 250 million women are infected with human papilloma virus (HPV). It has also been estimated that almost 900,000 pregnant women are infected with syphilis.[43] Females in sub-Saharan Africa have a burden of disease from STIs, other than HIV, that is three to five times higher than the burden that females face in the other World Bank regions.[43]

The risk factors for a woman getting an STI are well known and include young age when engaging in sexual relations, often because of child marriage, especially in Asia and sub-Saharan Africa; multiple sexual partners; sex with high-risk partners, including partners considerably older than the woman; and inability or unwillingness to use a condom. The use of alcohol and drugs is also associated with unprotected sex, as is unequal power between a woman and a man who are engaging in sexual relations.[44]

Sexually transmitted infections other than HIV that are not treated in a timely and appropriate manner can have a number of long-lasting effects on the health of women. These include pelvic inflammatory disease, chronic pain, ovarian abscesses, ectopic pregnancies, and infertility.[45] When pregnant women cannot get STIs treated in appropriate and timely ways, it can lead to fetal wastage, stillbirths, low birthweight babies, eye and lung damage in babies, and congenital abnormalities.[45]

Violence and Sexual Abuse Against Women

Violence and sexual abuse against women occur with remarkable frequency throughout the world. Violence is usually episodic, it is often not reported, and it is often associated with sexual abuse.[46] Sexual abuse can include rape, sexual assault, sexual molestation, sexual harassment, and incest.[47] It is very hard to get reliable data on violence and sexual abuse against women. WHO estimated that in 2018, "30 percent of women have been subjected to physical and/or sexual violence by an intimate partner or non-partner."[48,49] In addition, there have been a number of conflicts in which rape has been used systematically as a "weapon of war."[50]

It appears that violence against females is associated with factors such as young age of the male partner, a history of violence of the male partner, low socioeconomic status of the male and female involved, proximity to drugs or alcohol, social isolation, and gender inequality. The likelihood of violence is heightened in conflict and post-conflict situations.[49]

The Costs and Consequences of Ill Health Among Females

The costs of women's health problems are very substantial. In many societies, women are the primary caregivers to children, and when the health of the mother suffers, there is often a negative effect on the health of the children as well. In addition, women play important economic roles in many families, and the morbidity, disability, and mortality associated with particular problems of women's health have substantial economic implications.

Women are stigmatized by a variety of communicable diseases as well, such as TB, HIV/AIDS, and some of the neglected tropical diseases. There are also exceptional economic costs related to women's nutritional and health conditions, but these are not often given the attention they deserve. The costs of violence against women, especially in low-income countries, have not been studied carefully, but they are substantial. A study in Chile, for example, suggested that the costs of domestic violence were equal to 2% of Chile's gross domestic product (GDP). A similar study in Nicaragua indicated that such violence cost 1.6% of GDP.[47]

The economic costs of maternal health conditions are also high but not well documented. They also often fail to take account of morbidity associated with maternal health and not just mortality. These morbidities can seriously constrain women's productivity both in and outside of the home. They can also significantly reduce the income that women can earn. When a woman dies a premature maternal death, the economic losses are substantial, given the many years that the woman could have engaged in care of her family and worked inside and outside of the home. In addition, the death of a mother will likely damage the future prospects for economic well-being and economic contributions of any children who survive her. Similarly, depression in women also has high economic costs.

Addressing the Health of Females

Some countries, such as Sri Lanka, have been able to improve the health of women at relatively low levels of expenditure by making wise choices about investments in health and education. These included increasing female education, providing widespread access to midwives, and ensuring adequate backup for the midwives at hospitals.

The quest for universal health coverage in an increasing number of countries should also enhance the health of females. Improving the health of females in the future will also require that health systems provide a cost-effective package of services, including nutrition, family planning, prenatal care, deliveries attended by skilled healthcare providers, emergency transportation of women who are having complicated labors, and emergency obstetric services of appropriate quality at a hospital. A number of countries are now undertaking a variety of efforts, including incentive programs, to try to increase the demand for such services and the supply of these services at an appropriate level of quality.

In the long run, it will be important to change the gender roles that favor males, promote the education and empowerment of females, promote their prospects for earning income, and educate communities to better understand the health conditions that females face and the measures that can be taken to address them. Most countries also need to pay more attention to the overall health of females, and measures to reduce in cost-effective and fair ways the leading burdens of disease that females face, including the noncommunicable diseases and mental health disorders of importance to the health of females.

The Health of Under Five Children

Introduction

This section is about children under five years of age, largely in low- and middle-income countries.

It does not discuss **stillbirths**, which readers can review, for example, in materials from WHO[51] and *The Lancet* series that extensively covered stillbirths.[52] Early childhood development is also central to the well-being of children. However, it, too, is beyond the scope of this book, and readers can explore this further in the 2016 *Lancet* series on early childhood development.[53]

As one considers the health of young children, it is critical to remember that a range of interventions, across sectors, is needed to ensure that young children develop to their full biological and intellectual potential. It is also important to remember that without these interventions, a substantial portion of young children, especially in low- and middle-income countries, will never achieve their full potential.

The Importance of Child Health

There are a number of reasons why the health of young children is so important. First, it has been estimated that about 5.2 million children under five years of age died in 2019. This is equal to over 14,000 children under five who died *each day* that year.[54] The second reason is that an overwhelming portion of these deaths is preventable. Young children, for example, almost never die in high-income countries[55] and it has been estimated that more than half of child deaths each year could be avoided through known, simple, and low-cost interventions.[55] Third, children have a special place in the global health agenda because they are so vulnerable. Their vulnerability also raises important ethical issues about the responsibility of adults to ensure the health and survival of children. Child health is also closely linked with poverty. If families had more income, they would have greater access to water and sanitation, health, education, and other social services that would also serve children well.

The Status of Health of Young Children

There has been substantial progress in reducing the number of under five children who die each year globally, with the numbers going from one in 11 children dying before reaching age five in 1990 to one in 27 in 2019.[56] However, some parts of the world have not made sufficient progress in enhancing child health. This has been especially true in parts of sub-Saharan Africa and South Asia.

Of the 5.2 million children under five who die each year, as noted above, 47% of the deaths take place in the **neonatal** period, 28% in the **post-neonatal period**, and 25% between the first and fourth years.[54]

The chances of survival for a newborn, an infant, and a young child vary greatly across different settings. The neonatal mortality rate in 2019 was three per 1,000 live births in high-income countries, but 27 in low-income countries. The infant mortality rate was four per 1,000 live births in high-income countries but 48 in low-income countries.[57] The under five child mortality rate was five per 1,000 live births in high-income countries but 68 in low-income countries.[58]

In addition, the rates of neonatal, infant, and child mortality often vary substantially within countries, often depending on family income and education, location, and ethnicity. In India, for example, infant mortality varies from seven per 1,000 live births in Kerala state to 48 per 1,000 in Madhya Pradesh state.[59] In the United States, infant mortality was four per 1,000 live births for a white child in the Baltimore Metro Area and 10.2 per 1,000 live births for an African American child.[60]

In the higher income countries, in which the rates of young child death are low, few children die and about 60% of the deaths will be among neonates. However, particularly in South Asia and sub-Saharan Africa, children face important risks of dying as neonates, between 29 days and 1 year, and between 1 year and 5 years.[57,58,61]

The Burden of Disease Among Young Children

The 10 leading causes of death of under five children are neonatal disorders, lower respiratory infections, diarrheal diseases, congenital defects, malaria, meningitis, whooping cough (pertussis), protein-energy malnutrition, STIs excluding HIV, and measles.[34]

It is important to note the significance of neonatal disorders and congenital defects among the leading causes of death. The prominence of STIs—mostly congenital syphilis–is also striking. In addition, protein-energy malnutrition, basically children who are not getting enough food, is disturbingly important. The other causes among the top 10 are all communicable diseases, three of which, whooping cough, measles, and some respiratory infections, are vaccine preventable.[34]

The Determinants of Young Child Health

The 10 leading risk factors for the death of children under five years of age are low birth weight and short gestation, child growth failure, particulate matter, unsafe water, unsafe sanitation, handwashing, suboptimal breastfeeding, secondhand smoke, high temperature, and vitamin A deficiency.[34] The extent to which many young children face risks related to nutrition is clear and about 45% of all deaths of children under five years of age are related to children being undernourished.[1]

The social determinants of health have a major impact on the health of young children. Poverty is a significant underlying factor of food security and of morbidity and mortality among children. The lack of education for females and mothers is another very important determinant of the health of young children. The failure of many governments to invest in water, sanitation, and hygiene is a major cause of the death of under-five children worldwide.

Addressing the Health of Under Five Children

There are well-known, proven, and cost-effective interventions for substantially reducing the deaths of neonates, infants, and young children. Their deaths do not stem from a failure of knowing what to do. Rather, they stem mostly from a failure to reach all children with these interventions.

The key interventions can be oriented in a life-course approach—those important before pregnancy; those during pregnancy, birth, and shortly after birth; those needed in the post-neonatal period; and those most important for the young child. The following will be among the most important interventions:

- Ensuring the health and proper nourishment of the mother
- Providing access to modern contraceptives, prenatal care, and micronutrient supplementation for the mother-to-be
- Prevention of mother-to-child transmission of HIV/AIDS
- Attendance at delivery by a skilled birth attendant and referral for emergency obstetric care if needed
- Appropriate care of the newborn, special measures for low birthweight babies, and referral if needed for illness
- Early and exclusive breastfeeding for six months
- Hygienic introduction of diverse complementary foods
- Childhood immunization
- Bed nets for malaria and regular drug administration for worms
- Oral rehydration for diarrhea and early diagnosis and treatment for pneumonia[62]

The Health of Adolescents and Young Adults

What Are Adolescents and Young Adults?

There is an important debate about what age groups should be considered when one examines the health of "adolescents." Traditionally, "adolescence" was considered the period between puberty and marriage and parenthood.[63] The World Health Organization (WHO) considers adolescents to be people between 10 and 19 years of age.[64] Nonetheless, the endpoints of this period are not as clear as they were earlier. They also vary by cultural groups. Thus, the most recent study of importance on "adolescents" covered the age range of 10 to 24 years.[65]

There is little debate, however, about the importance of disaggregating this age range into several different groups if one is to get the best possible understanding of the health of "young people" across their life course. With this in mind, the 10- to 24-year period is broken down into three groups:

- 10–14: Early adolescence
- 15–19: Older adolescence
- 20–24: Young adulthood

The health of adolescents and young adults is critical to the global health agenda. Adolescents and young adults constitute an important part of the population in all countries. In addition, the health of adolescents and young adults is central to preserving the gains made in child health. It is also central to laying a solid foundation for the health of future adults.[65]

A specific focus on the health of adolescents and young adults is also essential because adolescents and young adults are neither children nor fully mature adults and because adolescence and young adulthood is a time of important biological and psychological change.[65]

The Burden of Disease Among Adolescents and Young Adults

Adolescents and young adults have a unique burden of disease. Early adolescents, especially in low- and middle-income countries, continue to fall ill and die from preventable or treatable communicable diseases, such as HIV/AIDS, malaria, diarrhea, pneumonia, and TB. Road injuries and drowning are also important causes of death in this group.[34] By contrast, in high-income countries, the leading causes of death among this group are road injuries, self-harm, congenital defects, a number of cancers, interpersonal violence, and pneumonia.[34]

The leading causes of death among adolescents 15 to 19 years of age in low-income countries include HIV/AIDS, road injuries, maternal disorders, TB, and diarrheal disease. Malaria, interpersonal violence, self-harm, and meningitis are also among the top 10 causes of death in this group.[34] There is a substantial shift in the burden in the same age group in high-income countries. Here, the leading causes of death are road injuries, self-harm, interpersonal violence, drug-use disorders, cancer, drowning, and falls.[34]

Group I causes continue to be important even among the 20 to 24-year-old age group. In low-income countries, the leading causes of death for this group will be road injuries, HIV/AIDS, TB, maternal disorders, and interpersonal violence. Malaria, self-harm, pneumonia, and meningitis complete the 10 leading causes of death in this group. The leading causes of death in this age group in high-income countries are exclusively noncommunicable causes and injuries: road injuries, self-harm, drug-use disorders, interpersonal violence, and falls.[34]

The risk factors for the communicable diseases that affect adolescents and young adults include, among other things, unsafe sex, unsafe water, poor hygiene, and poor nutrition. Early pregnancy is also an important risk factor for maternal morbidity and mortality. Particulate matter, alcohol use, and iron deficiency, particularly among females, are also key risk factors.[34] There is a substantial shift in risk factors, however, as one moves to high-income countries. For these countries, the leading risk factors include drug use, alcohol use, occupational injury, high body mass index, high-fasting plasma glucose, intimate partner violence, and kidney dysfunction.[34]

Social determinants of health, such as poverty, abuse, living in rural areas, poor family educational attainment, and gender discrimination are also key to understanding the burden of disease among adolescents and young adults. Peer relationships, living with conflict or the aftermath of disasters, and having few economic options are important determinants of the health and well-being of adolescents and young adults and whether they engage in tobacco use, alcohol abuse, unsafe sex, risky driving, or suffer from mental health issues.[65]

The five leading causes of DALYs for adolescents and young adults include skin diseases for all of the groups; self-harm for almost all of the age groups; road injuries and interpersonal violence for males; migraines, anxiety disorders, depressive disorders and dietary iron deficiency for females; and the continuing importance of HIV/AIDS for 10- to 14-year-old females and 15- to 19-year-old males.[34]

As we would expect, mortality rates rise as one goes from early adolescence to young adulthood. As we would also expect, mortality rates vary by region and country income groups. The lower the income level of the country, in general, the higher the mortality rate of any age group.[65]

Economic and Social Consequences of Health Issues Among Adolescents and Young Adults

Health issues among adolescents and young adults have profound consequences socially and economically. First, maintaining the health of adolescents and young adults is central to maintaining the gains that have occurred in the health of young children. More and more children are living longer and healthier lives as progress has been made, among other things, against vaccine-preventable diseases and malaria. This progress can be undone if adolescents and young adults face important health issues that take their lives away or lead to major illness or disability.

Second, the health of adolescents and young adults and behaviors in which they engage set a foundation for their health as adults. Adolescent pregnancy can diminish the chances that a girl will complete schooling or that her child will become a well-educated, healthy, and productive adult. Obesity during adolescence or young adulthood, for example, can have a permanent effect on the health and productivity of an adult. Most people who take up smoking tobacco, drinking alcohol, and using illegal drugs start such behaviors in adolescence, and these behaviors are difficult to stop as adults.

Other burdens of disease among adolescents and young adults also have substantial costs. The social and economic costs of HIV/AIDS are well known, and adolescent girls are among those at greatest risk of being infected with HIV. Tuberculosis is a major cause of morbidity and death among adolescents in Africa, and TB leads to months of lost work, even if treated effectively. Road traffic injuries, the leading cause of death among adolescents and young adults globally, can lead to substantial and long-lasting disabilities, as well as many years of life lost. Mental health issues often start in adolescence, go on for much or all of a person's life, and have enormous social and economic costs to individuals, their families, and societies.

Addressing the Health of Adolescents and Young Adults

There are a number of measures that can be taken to address the key health issues that adolescents and young adults face. At the broadest levels of society, it will be important to promote a good quality education to the secondary level for females as well as males. Investing in water, sanitation, and hygiene will also be fundamental. Economic policies that encourage job creation and productive employment for the large numbers of adolescents and young adults who will enter the job market will also be essential.[65]

Health systems can take a number of institutional steps to better address the health needs of adolescents and young adults as well. They need to train their staff to pay attention to the unique burdens of disease and needs of these groups. They need to improve their collection of data that is specific to adolescents and young adults as well. It will also be important that specific health programs, such as for TB or HIV, focus particular attention on adolescents and young adults, on the risk factors for becoming infected with active TB disease or with HIV, and on measures that could be taken to reduce the specific risks for these diseases that adolescents and young adults face. Moving to universal health coverage can also help to reduce the barriers that many adolescents and young adults face in accessing health services, as would ensuring that such health services are friendly to these groups.[65]

Other specific interventions could also be made to reduce the burden of disease among adolescents and young adults. Improving licensing requirements for driving, taking a stepwise approach to adolescent driving, and stricter enforcement of drunk driving laws can reduce road traffic injuries among these groups. Keeping girls in school longer, improving knowledge about reproductive health and family planning, and enhancing access to family planning and maternal health services could reduce the burden of reproductive health issues among adolescents and young adults. Taking a community-based approach to mental health issues, with specific attention to adolescents and young adults, psychosocial support, and referral for difficult cases, could help to reduce the high burden of mental health conditions and suicide among adolescents and young adults.[65]

Discussion Questions

1. What are the most important nutritional concerns for the health of young children in low- and middle-income countries and what can be done to address them?
2. In what ways can we say that "being born female is dangerous to your health?"
3. Why do approximately 5 million under-five children die globally each year and what can be done in the short and medium term to reduce such deaths?
4. What approaches can be taken to reduce the burden of mental health disorders in adolescents and young adults, especially in places where there are few medically trained mental health professionals?
5. In what ways are intersectoral approaches needed to enhance the health of young children?

References

1. Black RE, Victora CG, Walker SP, et al. Maternal and child undernutrition and overweight in low-income and middle-income countries. *Lancet*. 2013;382(9890):427–451.
2. Singh AS, Mulder C, Twisk JW, van Mechelen W, Chinapaw MJ. Tracking of childhood overweight into adulthood: a systematic review of the literature. *Obes Rev*. 2008;9(5): 474–488.
3. Hunt, JM. (2002). Reversing Productivity Losses from iron deficiency: The economic case. *Journal of Nutrition*, 132(Suppl. 4):794S–801S
4. World Health Organization. Malnutrition. Key facts. 2020A. Retrieved from https://www.who .int/news-room/fact-sheets/detail/malnutrition
5. World Health Organization. Low birth weight data by World Bank Income Group. 2019A. Retrieved from https://apps.who.int/gho/data/view.main-eu.LBWWBINCOMEGROUPv ?lang=en
6. The World Bank. Low-birthweight babies (% of births). nd, A. Retrieved March 16, 2021 from https://data.worldbank.org/indicator/SH.STA.BRTW.ZS?name_desc=false
7. The World Bank. Prevalence of stunting, height for age (% of children under 5). nd, B. Retrieved March 16, 2021 from https://data.worldbank.org/indicator/SH.STA.STNT.ZS
8. The World Bank. Prevalence of wasting, weight for height (% of children under 5). nd, C. Retrieved March 16, 2021 from https://data.worldbank.org/indicator/SH.STA.WAST.ZS
9. World Health Organization. Obesity and overweight. Key facts. 2020B. Retrieved from https://www.who.int/news-room/fact-sheets/detail/obesity-and-overweight
10. World Health Organization. Prevalence of obesity among adults, BMI ≥ 30, (age-standardized estimate). 2017A. Retrieved from https://www.who.int/data/gho/data/indicators/indicator -details/GHO/prevalence-of-obesity-among-adults-bmi-=-30-(age-standardized-estimate)-(-)
11. World Health Organization. Micronutrients. nd, A. Retrieved March 16, 2021, from https:// www.who.int/health-topics/micronutrients#tab=tab_1
12. The World Bank. Prevalence of anemia among children (% of children under 5). nd, D. Retrieved from https://data.worldbank.org/indicator/SH.ANM.CHLD.ZS
13. The World Bank. Prevalence of anemia among women of reproductive age (% of women ages 15-49). nd, E. Retrieved from https://data.worldbank.org/indicator/SH.ANM.ALLW.ZS
14. Victora CG, Christian P, Vidaletti LP, Gatica-Domínguez G, Menon P, Black RE. Revisiting maternal and child undernutrition in low-income and middle-income countries: variable progress towards an unfinished agenda. *Lancet*. 2021;397(10282):1388–1399. https://doi .org/10.1016/S0140-6736(21)00394-9
15. Malik V, Hu F. Obesity prevention. In: *Disease Control Priorities*. 3rd ed. *Cardiovascular, Respiratory, and Related Disorders*. Prabhakaran D, Anand S, Gaziano T, Mbanya J, Wu Y, Nugent R, eds. Washington, DC: World Bank; 2018: 5.
16. UNICEF. (2006). *Progress for children. A report card on nutrition, No. 4*. Retrieved from http:// www.unicef.org/progressforchildren/2006n4/index_undernutrition.html

17. GP Notebook. *Xerophthalmia*. Retrieved from http://www.gpnotebook.co.uk/simplepage .cfm?ID=664403984 nd.

18. Caulfield LE, Richard SA, Rivera JA, Musgrove P, Black RE. Stunting, wasting, and micronutrient disorders. In Jamison JG, Breman AR, Measham AR, et al. (eds.), *Disease control priorities in developing countries* (2nd ed., pp. 551–567). New York, NY: Oxford University Press: 2006.

19. World Health Organization. Global action plan for the prevention and control of noncommunicable diseases 2013–2020. 2013A. Retrieved from http://apps.who.int/iris /bitstream/10665/94384/1/9789241506236_eng.pdf

20. UNICEF Canada. Malnutrition. nd. Retrieved March 16, 2021 from https://www.unicef.ca/en /malnutrition

21. World Bank. 2006. Repositioning nutrition as central to development: a strategy for large-scale action. Washington, DC. © World Bank. https://openknowledge.worldbank.org/handle /10986/7409 License: CC BY 3.0 IGO.

22. International Food Policy Research Institute. *Global nutrition report 2014: Actions and accountability to accelerate the world's progress on nutrition*. Washington, DC: 2014.

23. Griffiths M, Dicken K, Favin M. *Promoting the growth of children: what works: Rationale and guidance for programs*. Washington, DC: World Bank; 1996.

24. Levinson FJ, Bassett L. *Malnutrition is still a major contributor to child deaths*. Washington, DC: Population Reference Bureau; 2008.

25. Lofti M, Merx R, Naber P, Van der Heuvel P. *Micronutrient fortification of foods: Current prospectus, research and opportunities*. Ottawa, Ontario, Canada: International Agriculture Centre; 1996.

26. World Health Organization. Obesity and Overweight. 2020C. Retrieved from https://www .who.int/en/news-room/fact-sheets/detail/obesity-and-overweight

27. World Health Organization. Tackling NCDs: Best buys and other recommended interventions for the prevention and control of noncommunicable diseases. Geneva, Switzerland; 2017B.

28. European Commission. Collated information on salt reduction in the EU, 2008. 2008. Retrieved from https://ec.europa.eu/health/ph_determinants/life_style/nutrition/documents /compilation_salt_en.pdf

29. World Health Organization Regional Office for the Eastern Mediterranean. Nutrition. nd. Retrieved from http://www.emro.who.int/nutrition/strategy/policy-statement-and-recommended -actions-for-lowering-sugar-intake-and-reducing-prevalence-of-type-2-diabetes-and-obesity -in-the-eastern-mediterranean-region.html#:~:text=The%20policy%20is%20based%20 on,most%20appropriate%20long%2Dterm%20goal

30. World Health Organization. REPLACE trans fat. nd, B. Retrieved March 16, 2021 from https://www.who.int/teams/nutrition-and-food-safety/replace-transfat#:~:text=The %20REPLACE%20action%20package%20provides,heart%20disease%20mortality%20 and%20events

31. Pekka P, Pirjo P, Ulla U. Influencing public nutrition for non-communicable disease prevention: from community intervention to national programme—experiences from Finland. *Publ Health Nutr.* 2002;5(1a):245–251.

32. World Health Organization. Tackling NCDs: best buys and other recommended interventions for prevention and control of noncommunicable diseases. Geneva, Switzerland; 2017C.

33. Murphy EM. Being born female is dangerous for your health. *Am Psychol.* 2003;58(3): 205–210.

34. Institute of Health Metrics and Evaluation (IHME). GBD Compare: Viz Hub. nd. Retrieved from https://vizhub.healthdata.org/gbd-compare/

35. World Health Organization. Maternal mortality. 2019B. Retrieved from https://www.who.int /news-room/fact-sheets/detail/maternal-mortality

36. World Health Organization. Obstetric fistula. 2018B. Retrieved from https://www.who.int /news-room/facts-in-pictures/detail/10-facts-on-obstetric-fistula

37. Bearak J, Popinchalk A, Ganatra B, et al. Unintended pregnancy and abortion by income, region, and the legal status of abortion: estimates from a comprehensive model for 1990–2019. *Lancet Glob Health.* 2020;8(9):e1152–e1161. doi: 10.1016/S2214-109X(20) 30315-6

38. World Health Organization (WHO). Preventing unsafe abortion. 2020D. Retrieved from https://www.who.int/news-room/fact-sheets/detail/preventing-unsafeabortion#:~:text=Each %20year%20between%204.7%25%20%E2%80%93%2013.2,to%20unsafe%20abortion%20 (3).percenttext=Around%207%20million%20women%20are,of%20unsafe%20abortion %20(4)

39. World Health Organization. Female genital mutilation. 2018B. Retrieved from http://www .who.int/news-room/fact-sheets/detail/female-genital-mutilation

40. UNICEF. Female genital mutilation/cutting: A statistical overview and exploration of the dynamics of change. York, NY: UNICEF. 2014.

41. Kandala NB, Ezejimofor MC, Uthman OA, Komba P. Secular trends in the prevalence of female genital mutilation/cutting among girls: a systematic analysis. *BMJ Global Health*. 2018;3(5):e000549. doi: 10.1136/bmjgh-2017-000549

42. Glasier A, Gülmezoglu AM, Schmid GP, Moreno CG. Look PFV. Sexual and reproductive health: a matter of life and death. *Lancet*. 2006;368(9547):1595–1607.

43. World Health Organization. Sexually transmitted infections (STIs). 2013B. Retrieved from http://apps.who.int/iris/bitstream/10665/82207/1/WHO_RHR_13.02_eng.pdf

44. Buvinic M, Medici A, Fernandez E, Torres AC. Gender differentials in health. In: Jamison DT, Breman JG, Measham AR, et al., (eds). *Disease Control Priorities in Developing Countries*. 2nd edition. New York, NY: Oxford University Press; 2006:195–210.

45. WHO. *Sexually Transmitted Infections*. Retrieved from https://www.who.int/news-room/fact-sheets/detail/sexually-transmitted-infections-(stis) 2019.

46. Tinker A. A new agenda for women's health and nutrition. Washington, DC: The World Bank; 1994.

47. Rosenberg ML, Butchart A, Mercy J, Narasimhan V, Waters H, Marshall MS. Interpersonal violence. In: Jamison DT, Breman JG, Measham AR, et al., eds. *Disease Control Priorities in Developing Countries*. 2nd edition. New York, NY: Oxford University Press; 2006:755–770.

48. World Health Organization. Violence against women. 2021C. Retrieved from https://www .who.int/news-room/fact-sheets/detail/violence-against-women#:~:text=Globally%20as%20 many%20as%2038,sexual%20violence%20are%20more%20limited%20

49. World Health Organization. Violence against women. Retrieved from https://www.who.int /news-room/fact-sheets/detail/violence-against-women 2021D.

50. United Nations Human Rights Office of the High Commissioner. Rape: a weapon of war. nd. Retrieved from https://www.ohchr.org/en/newsevents/pages/rapeweaponwar.aspx

51. World health Organization. Stillbirth. nd. Retrieved from https://www.who.int/health-topics /stillbirth#tab=tab_

52. De Bernis L, Kinney MV, Stinbes W, et al. Ending preventable stillbirths. *Lancet*. 2016A;387(10019):703–716.

53. Advancing early childhood development: from science to scale. Lancet. 2016B. Retrieved from https://www.thelancet.com/series/ECD2016

54. World Health Organization. Children: reducing mortality (Fact sheet no. 178). 2018D. Retrieved from http://www.who.int/mediacentre/factsheets/fs178/en/

55. Bhutta ZA, Ahmed T, Black RE, Cousens S, Dewey K, Giugliani E. What works? Interventions for maternal and child undernutrition and survival. *Lancet*.2020;371(9610):417–440.

56. World Health Organization. Children: improving survival and well-being. 2020F. Retrieved from https://www.who.int/news-room/fact-sheets/detail/children-reducing-mortality#:~:text =In%202019%20an%20estimated%205.2,from%20preventable%20and%20treatable %20causes

57. The World Bank. Mortality rate, infant (per 1,000 live births). nd, G. Retrieved from https://data.worldbank.org/indicator/SP.DYN.IMRT.IN

58. World Bank Data. Mortality rate, under-5 (per 1,000 pive births). nd. Retrieved from https:// data.worldbank.org/indicator/SH.DYN.MORT

59. Census of India. Estimates of mortality indicators. 2018. Retrieved from https://censusindia .gov.in/vital_statistics/SRS_Report_2018/11.%20Chap%204-Estimates%20of%20Mortality %20Indicators-2018.pdf

60. Maryland Department of Health. Maryland Vital Statistics Infant Mortality in Maryland, 2018. 2019. Retrieved from https://health.maryland.gov/vsa/Documents/Infant_Mortality _Report_2018.pdf
61. World Bank|Data. Mortality rate, neonatal (per 1,000 live births). nd. Retrieved from https://data.worldbank.org/indicator/SH.DYN.NMRT
62. World Health Organization. Family and community practices that promote child survival, growth, and development: A review of the evidence. Geneva, Switzerland; 2004.
63. Sawyer SM, Afifi RA, Bearinger LH, et al. Adolescence: a foundation for future health. *Lancet.* 2012;379(9826):1630–1640.
64. World Health Organization (WHO). *Adolescent health.* Retrieved from https://www.who.int /topics/adolescent_health/en/ nd, C
65. World Health Organization (WHO). Health for the world's adolescents: a second chance in the second decade. Geneva, Switzerland; 2014. Retrieved from https://apps.who.int.adolescent /second-decade/

CHAPTER 6

Communicable Diseases

LEARNING OBJECTIVES

By the end of this chapter, the reader will be able to do the following:

- Review the burden of communicable diseases
- Discuss the determinants of selected communicable diseases, including emerging and re-emerging infectious diseases and antimicrobial resistance
- Review the costs and consequences of communicable diseases of importance
- Outline critical measures to address the leading communicable disease burdens in evidence-based, fair, and cost-effective ways

VIGNETTES

Henrietta was a 35-year-old Kenyan mother of four who lived in Mombasa. Over the last four months, Henrietta was barely able to digest her food, had frequent bouts of diarrhea, and had been losing weight. She worried about having AIDS. Henrietta went to a local clinic where she was tested and found to be HIV-positive. She had been infected by her husband, who was a long-distance truck driver.

Maria was 33 years old and lived in the mountains of Peru. For some time, she had not been feeling well. She often had a fever, was coughing a lot, and had night sweats. Maria had tuberculosis (TB) earlier and worried that she might have TB again. In fact, this time she had drug-resistant TB, which would be difficult and expensive to treat.

Wole was 4 years old and lived in southwestern Nigeria. He had flu-like symptoms, a fever, and a headache. His mother suspected he might have malaria but decided to treat him herself. In another few days, however, Wole was much sicker and lapsed into a coma. His mother rushed him to the local health center, but he died within a few hours. Unfortunately, Wole had the most virulent form of malaria.

The Importance of Communicable Diseases

Communicable diseases are immensely important to the global burden of disease. In 2019, they accounted for approximately 18% of all deaths globally and 26% of all disability-adjusted life years (DALYs). However, in low-income countries, they accounted for about 51% of all deaths and 58% of all DALYs.[1]

These diseases disproportionately affect the poor. Better-off people have the knowledge and income to protect themselves from diseases spread by unsafe water. They do not live in the crowded circumstances that can spread TB, and they also protect themselves as much as possible against malaria. In addition, they immunize their children against vaccine-preventable diseases at higher rates than poor people do.

Communicable diseases are also of enormous economic consequence. These diseases constrain the physical and mental development of infants and young children and reduce their future economic prospects. The impacts of HIV, TB, malaria, and the neglected tropical diseases on adult productivity are also exceptionally large. In addition, the direct and indirect costs of treatment for an infected person are often a substantial portion of their income.

Key Terms, Definitions, and Concepts

Key terms related to communicable diseases are defined in **Table 6-1**. A communicable disease is a disease that is transmitted from an animal to another animal, an animal to a human, a human to another human, or a human to an animal. Transmission

---

Table 6-1 Communicable Disease Definitions

Case—An individual with a particular disease.
Case fatality rate—The proportion of persons with a particular condition (cases) who die from that condition.
Control (disease control)—Reducing the incidence and prevalence of a disease to an acceptable level.
Elimination (of disease)—Reducing the incidence of a disease in a specific area to zero.
Emerging infectious disease—A newly discovered disease.
Eradication (of disease)—Termination of all cases of a disease and its transmission globally.
Parasite—An organism that lives in or on another organism and takes its nourishment from that organism.
Re-emerging infectious disease—An existing disease that has increased in incidence or has taken on new forms.

Data from Centers for Disease Control and Prevention (CDC). (nd). Epidemiology glossary. Retrieved from https://www.cdc .gov/reproductivehealth/data_stats/glossary.html; Dowdle, W. R. (1999). The principles of disease elimination and eradication. *Morbidity and Mortality Weekly Report*, 48(Suppl. 1):23–27. Retrieved from http://www.cdc.gov/mmwr/preview/mmwrhtml /su48a7.htm

can be direct, such as through respiratory means, or indirect through a vector, such as a mosquito in the case of malaria. Most people use the term **communicable disease** in a manner that is synonymous with **infectious disease**.

Communicable diseases can be spread in the following ways (examples of diseases spread in these ways are also cited): **foodborne**: salmonella, Escherichia coli; **waterborne**: cholera, rotavirus; **sexual** or **bloodborne**: hepatitis, HIV; **vector-borne**: malaria, onchocerciasis; **inhalation**: tuberculosis, influenza; **nontraumatic contact**: anthrax; and **traumatic contact**: rabies.

In addition, it is critical to understand the ways in which communicable diseases can be controlled. Examples are cited here, too, of diseases controlled in these ways:

- **Vaccination**: smallpox, polio, measles
- **Mass chemotherapy**: onchocerciasis, hookworm, lymphatic filariasis
- **Vector control**: malaria, dengue, yellow fever, onchocerciasis
- **Improved water, sanitation, hygiene**: diarrheal diseases
- **Improved care seeking, disease recognition**: diarrheal and respiratory diseases
- **Case management (treatment) and improved caregiving**: diarrheal disease, respiratory disease, HIV/AIDS, TB
- **Case surveillance, reporting, and containment**: avian influenza, meningitis, cholera
- **Behavioral change**: HIV, sexually transmitted infections, Guinea worm, Ebola virus

A final concept of exceptional importance when discussing communicable diseases is the concept of **drug resistance**. This refers to the extent to which infectious and parasitic agents develop an ability to resist drug treatment.

The Burden of Communicable Diseases

Broadly speaking, when we look at the burden of deaths and DALYs, we can say the following:

- The burden of communicable causes of death remains greatest in low-income countries.
- As country incomes rise, the share of deaths associated with communicable causes falls.
- In high-income countries, only a very small share of total deaths, mostly among the elderly, are caused by communicable diseases.

Globally, for all ages, two of the top 10 causes of death are communicable diseases: lower respiratory infections and diarrheal diseases. However, in lower-income countries, lower respiratory infections, diarrheal disease, malaria, tuberculosis, and HIV/AIDS are all among the 10 leading causes of death.[1]

Diarrheal disease is the only communicable disease in the top 10 causes of DALYs globally for all ages. However, lower respiratory infections, diarrheal diseases, malaria, HIVAIDS, and tuberculosis are all among the top five causes of DALYs for lower-income countries.[1] Communicable diseases remain among the most important causes of death of children under five years of age globally. Lower respiratory infections, diarrheal diseases, malaria, meningitis, whooping cough, sexually transmitted infections, and measles are all among the top 10 causes of death in this age group globally.[1]

The relative importance of specific communicable diseases to the burden of disease varies by region. HIV/AIDS is of particular importance in sub-Saharan Africa, as is malaria. The neglected tropical diseases are also much more important in sub-Saharan Africa than in any other region.[1]

The Costs and Consequences of Communicable Diseases

The economic and social costs of communicable diseases are high. First, these diseases constrain the health and development of infants and children and can impact their schooling and their productivity as adults. Second, stigma and discrimination against people with HIV, tuberculosis (TB), and a variety of other debilitating communicable diseases, such as leprosy and lymphatic filariasis, are strong. Third, adults who suffer from the diseases discussed in this chapter suffer substantial losses in productivity and income. Fourth, families spend considerable amounts of money trying to treat these illnesses. Fifth, high rates of communicable diseases in any country reduce investments in that country's development. Finally, as noted earlier, emerging and re-emerging infectious diseases can have enormous economic consequences as we have seen recently with COVID-19.

The Leading Burdens of Communicable Diseases

The sections that follow examine emerging and re-emerging infectious diseases and antimicrobial resistance, HIV, TB, malaria, diarrhea, and neglected tropical diseases.

Emerging and Re-emerging Infectious Diseases and Antimicrobial Resistance

The Burden of Emerging and Re-emerging Infectious Diseases

Throughout human history, new diseases have appeared periodically. The first recorded epidemic of the bubonic plague was in the 6th century. More recently, new diseases have emerged, such as the Ebola virus in 1976, HIV in the 1980s, severe acute respiratory syndrome (SARS) in the 1990s, and H5N1 influenza, commonly called "bird flu," which first appeared in humans in 2003. A novel coronavirus appeared in 2019. These new diseases are referred to as **emerging infectious diseases**.[2,3] Some of these diseases have infected only a limited number of people, while others have infected hundreds of millions of people.

Even as new diseases have emerged, some existing diseases have spread more widely in areas in which they had already been present, have spread to places in which they had not appeared before, or have taken on new forms. These diseases are referred to as **re-emerging infectious diseases**.[2,3] In recent years, there have been outbreaks of a number of re-emerging infectious diseases, including West Nile virus in the Western Hemisphere and Ebola in West Africa.

Resistant forms of disease can emerge or re-emerge when bacteria, parasites, and viruses are altered through mutation, natural selection, or the exchange of genetic material among strains and species.[4] The development of resistance is a natural phenomenon; however, it can be sped up by human action and a failure to address it in timely and effective ways.

Emerging and re-emerging infectious diseases and antimicrobial resistance are excellent examples of critical global health issues. They can arise anywhere and at any time. They can spread, sometimes rapidly, within and across countries. Different countries, with the help of various international organizations and networks, have to work together in technically sound ways if these issues are to be addressed effectively.

In fact, the threat of emerging and re-emerging infectious diseases is continuous and has been called "a perpetual challenge."[2] One study revealed that approximately 60% of these events were related to **zoonoses**—the spread of infection from animals to humans. The study also indicated that most of those events came from wildlife, and that wildlife was related to an increasing share of emerging and re-emerging infections over time. About 23% were related to vector-borne diseases that are spread by arthropods, such as mosquitoes, ticks, or fleas.[5]

The problem of drug resistance is also substantial. It is estimated that in 2018, there were 484,000 cases of TB globally that were resistant to the most effective first-line drug, rifampicin. In addition, about 187,000 of these cases were multidrug resistant, of which about 12,000 were extensively drug resistant.[6] There is also resistance to all of the drugs that treat malaria.

The most important factors that contribute to the emergence and re-emergence of infectious diseases include climate and weather, changing ecosystems, economic development and land use, human demographics and behavior, international travel and commerce, breakdown of public health measures, and war and famine.[7]

The factors that contribute to the development of drug resistance include[8,9] the increasing use of antibiotics; poor prescribing and dispensing practices; inappropriate use of the drugs; failure of patients to take appropriate doses of drugs; the use of counterfeit or poor-quality drugs; too much use of antibiotics in agriculture, cattle and poultry raising, and fish farming; and weak health systems with poor laboratory capacity to diagnose disease and test for drug susceptibility.

Some of the factors that might contribute to the more rapid spread of resistant forms of disease include weak infection control in healthcare settings, poor sanitation and hygiene, and a lack of surveillance.[8,10,11]

The Consequences of Emerging and Re-emerging Infectious Diseases

The costs of emerging and re-emerging diseases have varied considerably and have sometimes been very large. The plague in India in 1994 had an estimated cost of $1.7 billion. The economic costs of the mad cow outbreak in the United Kingdom were around $30 billion.[12]

It is important to note that these costs are not in proportion to deaths from these events. Between 1990 and 1998, for example, only 41 people died in the United Kingdom of mad cow disease.[3] Although SARS generated great fears, only

774 deaths were caused by this disease.[12] A substantial number of deaths *are* associated with some outbreaks, such as the West Africa Ebola outbreak. Yet, the economic costs of some of these events often appear to be related to the fear of possible spread rather than the actual morbidity and mortality caused by the disease. However, as we have seen with the coronavirus outbreak that began in 2019, diseases can have exceptional social and economic costs. Some of these may be direct costs, like the costs of hospitalization. Other costs are indirect and relate, for example, to the social costs of school closings and of economic disruption related to measures taken to control an outbreak.

The costs and consequences of drug resistance are also very high. A recent WHO report suggested, for example, that the median cost among 30 countries of treating multidrug-resistant TB was almost six times as high as the cost of treating drug-susceptible TB.[13] In addition, people are sicker longer and sometimes die from resistant strains of disease as health providers try to find drugs to which these diseases are susceptible. Moreover, the use of some drugs actually encourages the development of resistance to other drugs, making it harder to treat some conditions.[8]

Addressing Emerging and Re-emerging Infectious Diseases

The foundation for strengthening the capacity to address emerging and re-emerging infectious diseases has to focus on "highly sensitive national surveillance systems, public health laboratories that can rapidly detect outbreaks caused by emerging and re-emerging infections, and mechanisms that permit timely containment."[3] This must also be coupled with the willingness of countries to share information about disease outbreaks in a timely manner with other countries. There is also a need for global coordination of these efforts.

Disease surveillance is based on Global Outbreak Alert and Response Network (GOARN), a network of existing disease surveillance networks established in 2000.[14] The World Health Organization (WHO) published an updated version of the International Health Regulations (IHR) in 2005.[14] The IHR laid out a framework that is intended to guide national and global efforts at strengthening surveillance capacity and the national and global capacity to respond to outbreaks. In 2014, the global community established a new program for cooperation to help address emerging and re-emerging infectious diseases more effectively, the Global Health Security Agenda.[15]

Global efforts to address drug resistance have been inadequate. There has been some progress in addressing resistance on a disease-by-disease basis, such as efforts to better diagnose, track, and treat drug-resistant TB or drug-resistant malaria. There have also been countries, particularly in Europe, that have sought to reduce the use of antibiotics in both humans and animals. Nonetheless, the world has failed to establish a well-coordinated mechanism that can work across countries and diseases to address, in a coherent, timely, and effective manner, the factors that drive the development of drug resistance.[8]

In 2015, WHO published a Global Action Plan on Antimicrobial Resistance.[16] The plan aims to raise awareness of the problem, strengthen the evidence base for action, reduce the incidence of infection, optimize the use of antimicrobials in human and animal health, and develop the economic case for action against antimicrobial resistance. The 2018 WHO surveillance report on antibiotic use, however, reports continuing insufficient progress in meeting some of the key aims of the plan.[17]

The problem of drug resistance is also compounded by the limited number of new anti-infective drugs that are under development and the speed with which even new drugs become subject to resistance.[8] In addition, there has been insufficient research and development for drugs to combat some of the most important burdens of disease for the poor in low- and middle-income countries, including those for which there is increasing resistance. Until recently, for example, almost all of the existing TB drugs were at least 40 years old. WHO, among others, has recently sought to encourage investment in new antibiotics by establishing a working group on "high priority pathogens."[18]

A final note should be added about **pandemic preparedness**, which refers to the ability to effectively deal with a global outbreak of disease. An important question on this score is the extent to which individual countries and the global community as a whole are "ready" to identify and respond to the emergence of a pandemic influenza or other pandemic pathogen, such as the novel coronavirus that began to spread worldwide in 2019. There is widespread agreement that there are major gaps in pandemic preparedness and that many countries and the world as a whole are *not* adequately prepared to detect, prevent, or respond to a major global emergency.[19-21]

HIV/AIDS

The Burden of HIV/AIDS

In 2019, HIV affected 38 million people worldwide. That year an additional 1.7 million were newly infected with HIV, and 690,000 people died from it.[22]

HIV is a virus that can be spread in several different ways: unprotected sex, primarily vaginal and anal intercourse; mother-to-child transmission during childbirth or through breastfeeding; blood, including by transfusion, needle sharing, or accidental needle stick; and transplantation of infected tissue or organs. Being an uncircumcised male increases the risk of acquiring HIV. Females are also at greater biological and social risk than males of being infected with HIV. Having a sexually transmitted disease also increases the risk of HIV infection.

The efficiency with which the virus is transmitted varies. The virus is spread most efficiently from exposure to infected blood products and through the sharing of infected needles.[23] The efficiency of transmission is also relatively high from sharing needles with an HIV-infected person. Sexual transmission depends on the type of sexual act and whether the HIV-positive person is male or female. Male-to-female transmission is higher than female-to-male transmission. The risk of unprotected receptive anal intercourse is about 30 times greater than it is for receptive or insertive vaginal intercourse.[23]

As their disease reaches a fairly advanced state, HIV-positive people who are not on antiretroviral therapy may fall ill with TB, herpes infections, a variety of cancers, and an array of significant communicable diseases such as toxoplasmosis and cryptococcal meningitis. The latter has become a major killer of those infected with HIV.[24]

It is estimated that about 76 million people have been infected with HIV since the start of the epidemic, and about 33 million people have died from AIDS-related deaths since then. AIDS-related deaths have declined by 60% since the peak of the epidemic.[22] In sub-Saharan Africa, 75% of new infections in people aged 15 to 24 years are women, and women in sub-Saharan Africa are twice as likely as men to be living with HIV.[22]

The prevalence of HIV varies considerably by region and by country. The WHO region with the highest rate of new infections in 2019 was Africa. It was followed, although with much lower rates of incidence, by the Americas and South-East Asia. Eswatini, formerly known as Swaziland, had the highest HIV/AIDS prevalence rate in 2019, at 27%. The next highest rates were found in Lesotho, 23%; Botswana, at 21%; and South Africa, at 19%.[25]

The Global Burden of Disease Study 2019 indicated that HIV/AIDS was the 17th leading cause of death for all age groups globally, but the third leading cause globally for those aged 15 to 49 years. It was the third leading cause in sub-Saharan Africa among all age groups but the leading cause for those 15 to 49 years. HIV/AIDS was the 11th leading cause of DALYs globally for all age groups and the fifth leading cause for sub-Saharan Africa. For the 15- to 49-year-old age group, HIV/AIDS was the second leading cause of DALYs globally and the leading cause in sub-Saharan Africa.[1]

HIV Treatment

There is a global commitment to the following goals for those who are HIV-positive:

- Ninety percent of those with HIV are aware of their status.
- Ninety percent of those who have been diagnosed are placed on antiretroviral therapy.
- Ninety percent of those on therapy have an undetectable **viral load**.[26]

Meeting these targets is central to the global plan to reduce new HIV infections to 500,000 in 2020 and 200,000 in 2030.[27] UNAIDS estimated that in 2019, 81% of HIV-positive people knew their status, 82% of them were on antiretroviral therapy, and 88% of them had a suppressed viral load.[27]

The Costs and Consequences of HIV

HIV has significant social and economic consequences, especially in high-prevalence countries in sub-Saharan Africa, which go beyond its impact on morbidity and mortality. HIV affects family cohesion, business, trade, labor, the armed forces, agricultural production, education systems, governance, public services, and even national security.[28]

Another important consequence of HIV is the creation of a large number of orphans, defined as a child who has lost one or both parents to the disease. UNICEF estimated in 2019 that about 13.8 million children aged 0 to 17 years of age were "AIDS orphans."[29]

Like a number of other communicable diseases, HIV is a highly stigmatized condition. HIV, however, has a special stigma because people in many societies believe that people acquire HIV by engaging in behaviors that society does not sanction, such as men having sex with men, commercial sex work, or injecting drug use.

Understanding the notion of stigma and discrimination against people with HIV/AIDS is central to understanding the epidemic.

There has been enormous progress in making antiretroviral therapy widely available and at much cheaper prices. Today, the annual cost of therapy for first-line drugs is below $100 for low-income countries.[30] Although these costs are dramatically lower than before, it will be difficult for low-income countries with high HIV prevalence to support the costs of such treatment without considerable and sustained external assistance.[31]

Addressing the Burden of HIV/AIDS

Despite considerable efforts, there is not yet either a preventive or therapeutic vaccine for HIV. In the absence of such a vaccine, halting the spread of HIV will have to focus on the prevention of new infections. Several countries had early prevention efforts that were considered successful, such as Cambodia, Thailand, and Uganda. Such successes have consistently been associated with a number of factors, such as sustained political leadership at the highest levels; involvement of a broad range of civil society efforts, including opinion leaders and religious leaders; broad-based programs to change social norms in the population; open communication about HIV/AIDS and related sexual matters; and programs to reduce stigma and discrimination.[32]

In addition, we also know that to be successful, efforts to address HIV/AIDS need to include the following: good epidemic surveillance; information, education, and communication; voluntary counseling and testing; condom promotion; screening and treatment for sexually transmitted infections; prevention of mother-to-child transmission through antiretroviral treatment and avoiding pregnancy; voluntary male medical circumcision; interventions that target populations that transmit the virus from high-risk to low-risk populations; and prevention of bloodborne transmission through blood safety, harm reduction for injecting drug users, and universal precautions in healthcare settings.[27]

These efforts should also be linked with pre-exposure prophylaxis in selected populations. Effort to address HIV/AIDS were intended to ensure by 2020 the following: 90% of the people with HIV will know their HIV status, 90% of those with HIV will be receiving antiretroviral therapy, and 90% of those being treated will have suppressed viral loads.[27]

At the same time, countries need to continue to address stigma and discrimination against HIV-affected people. In addition, prevention efforts have to include a combination of approaches, what is called "combination prevention,"[33] with different weight given to different activities, depending on the nature of the epidemic. These efforts will have to combine three different types of approaches: biomedical, behavioral, and structural. **Biomedical** refers to approaches such as male medical circumcision, the treatment of other sexually transmitted infections, and antiretroviral therapy. **Behavioral** refers to efforts to change people's behavior so they have less risk of becoming infected with HIV. **Structural** refers to societal elements that may predispose a person to the risk of HIV. In this case, for example, adolescent girls who are poor may engage in "transactional sex" in exchange for financial help in order to support themselves, their schooling, or their families. Yet, if mechanisms can be put in place that can assist the girls in raising the funds needed for these matters, one might be able to reduce transactional sex and thereby reduce the number of those infected with HIV.

There has also been increasing attention paid to trying to stem mother-to-child transmission of HIV. The most cost-effective measure to reduce mother-to-child transmission of HIV is to avoid unwanted pregnancies of HIV-positive women through contraception. Providing antiretroviral therapy to pregnant women infected with HIV is also cost-effective.[34] If done properly, it can essentially eliminate mother-to-child transmission, whereas in the absence of such treatment, approximately one-third of HIV-positive pregnant women will give birth to a baby who is HIV-positive.[35] There is evidence that circumcised males are 40 to 60% less likely to be infected with HIV than uncircumcised males.[36] A number of voluntary medical male circumcision efforts are now underway as a component of HIV/AIDS prevention activities. Kenya has made important progress in this area, and it will be important to learn from this and other experiences about the most cost-effective approaches to scaling up voluntary male medical circumcision in different settings.[37]

Ensuring that the blood supply is safe and free of HIV, among other infectious agents, is cost-effective and must be a high priority in all settings.

As noted earlier, there has been substantial progress in low- and middle-income countries in placing HIV-infected people on antiretroviral therapy. This is not only important to ensure better health of the HIV-affected person but also to suppress their viral load so that they do not transmit HIV to others.

Overall, effective HIV/AIDS therapy depends on individuals accessing counseling and testing, a definitive HIV test, a clinical diagnosis of the patient, a laboratory assessment of the individual's immune status with a viral load test, patient adherence to their drug regimen, sound patient nutrition, and sound and continuous monitoring and evaluation of the patient.

Tuberculosis

The Burden of Tuberculosis

There were 10 million new TB cases in 2019, of which 820,000 were among people living with HIV. In 2019, 1.4 million people died of TB. Approximately 500,000 TB cases were resistant to rifampicin, the most effective first line drug, and 78% of those were multidrug resistant. The 2019 TB incidence rate per 100,000 population by WHO region was: Europe, 26; the Americas, 29; Western Pacific, 93; Eastern Mediterranean; 114; South-East Asia, 217; and Africa, 226.[38]

Most tuberculosis is caused by the bacteria *Mycobacterium tuberculosis*, which is spread through aerosol droplets. People breathe in the TB bacteria that is transmitted from other people who are ill with tuberculosis disease. Tuberculosis can affect all organs of the body, but in about 80% of the cases, the infection is in the lungs.[39,40]

However, zoonotic TB is another form of tuberculosis that affects humans. It is caused by *Mycobacterium bovis*, which is generally found in cattle (bovine TB) but can also be found in other animals. Most commonly, it is transmitted from infected food products, such as unpasteurized dairy products. This form of TB is often extrapulmonary and may be difficult to diagnose. This type of TB is also naturally resistant to one of the first-line drugs for *Mycobacterium tuberculosis*, making it harder to treat than that bacterium.[41]

To get TB (*Mycobacterium tuberculosis*), one has to be exposed to someone with the disease. The likelihood of exposure is greater if you are living with people with active pulmonary TB, especially under crowded circumstances, such as slum dwellings or prisons. Homeless people are also more susceptible to becoming ill with TB. Indeed, TB is generally thought of as a "disease of poverty."

An untreated person with active pulmonary TB can infect 10 to 15 people annually. About two-thirds of those with active TB disease will die of the disease if not treated properly. Pulmonary TB can be spread from person to person, but people with TB in other organs (extrapulmonary TB) generally do not spread TB. Active TB disease is characterized by a persistent cough for more than three weeks, decreased appetite, general weakness, and profuse night sweats.[39,40]

Not everyone infected with TB bacteria becomes sick with it. Rather, TB remains latent in the bodies of about 90% of those infected, and they will not develop active TB disease. People with latent TB do not spread TB to others. About one-third of the world's population is thought to be infected with TB. It is estimated that the infection will break down to cause active TB in approximately 10% of those people, especially if the person is immunocompromised.[39] This could occur because of malnutrition, HIV infection, use of immune-suppressing drugs, illness such as diabetes, or some cancers. Smoking and alcohol use are also risk factors for TB.[42]

The relationship between TB and HIV is a very important public health issue, as noted above. In addition to greatly increasing the risk of developing active TB disease, HIV is also associated with a higher proportion of TB that is not pulmonary, compared with TB that is not linked to HIV.[42]

WHO now recommends that initial diagnostic testing for anyone suspected of having TB be done with Xpert™ MTB/RIF. This test uses molecular techniques and can diagnose both TB and resistance to one of the first-line drugs for treatment, rifampicin, in less than 2 hours. Xpert MTB/RIF is more sensitive and more specific than sputum smear microscopy, which has been used traditionally for diagnosis of pulmonary TB and is still used in places that have not yet adopted the Xpert MTB/RIF tool.[43] Diagnosing TB in HIV-positive people and children may require other clinical diagnostic processes, as does extrapulmonary TB, that are not discussed here.[44,45]

Exposure and susceptibility are linked to males getting active TB disease more than females. However, there is variability in relative burden by sex in different age groups and in different settings.[46] Thus it is critical to note that TB is also a leading killer of women. About 900,000, or 9%, of the new cases of active TB were in people coinfected with HIV.[38]

There has been an increase in TB infections that are resistant to one or more TB drugs.[38] An underlying cause for the development of resistant forms of TB is the failure to complete TB treatment. However, it is also possible to be infected with drug-resistant TB directly from another person. Drug-resistant strains are found in many countries and are difficult and expensive to treat. Drug resistance is especially important in countries in which drug regulation and TB programs are weak or have fallen into disarray, such as Eastern Europe, and the greatest burdens of drug-resistant TB today are in Eastern Europe, China, and India.[38]

The incidence rate of TB varies considerably across countries and regions. In high-income countries, the incidence rate is generally below 10 per 100,000 population. By contrast, the highest burden countries generally have rates between 150 and 400 per 100,000. TB incidence has fallen globally but slowly, at a rate of approximately 2% per year. India, China, and Russia accounted for about half of all of the drug-resistant cases in the world.[13]

In the 2019 study of the global burden of disease, TB was the 13th most important cause of death worldwide for all age groups and both sexes, but it was the eighth leading cause in sub-Saharan Africa. However, for those 15 to 49 years of age in sub-Saharan Africa, TB was the second-leading cause of death. When we consider DALYs for the 15- to 49-year-old age group, TB was the second leading cause in sub-Saharan Africa and the fifth leading cause globally. Although TB kills substantially more men than women, TB is the eighth leading cause of death globally among women ages 15 to 49, and for men, TB is the seventh leading cause of death globally in this age group.[1]

The Costs and Consequences of TB

The cost of TB to families, communities, and countries is very high, given the large number of people who are sick with TB, the relatively long course of the illness, and the losses people face when they do have TB. A study of TB in India suggested that those sick with TB lost about 3 months of wages, spent an amount equal to about one-quarter of national income per capita on care and treatment, and took on debts to pay for this care that were equal to about 10% of per capita income.[47] There are also significant social costs. Because of the stigma associated with TB, females who fall ill with this disease in some parts of the world may be shunned by their families.

Addressing the Burden of TB

A vaccine for TB called Bacillus Calmette–Guérin (BCG) is a standard part of the Expanded Program of Immunization for Children. The vaccine reduces severe TB in children, but because children are not important transmitters of TB and due to variable efficacy of the vaccine in different settings, the vaccine has had little impact on the overall incidence or prevalence of TB.[48] Rather, the control of TB depends on effective treatment of active tuberculosis. In many respects, implementing a poor TB program is worse than having no TB program at all because a poor-quality TB program can give rise to drug-resistant TB by enabling the use of drugs without quality of care. Poor quality TB care can also lead to death in patients who should have been treated successfully.

WHO recommends a 6-month regimen for drug-susceptible disease that includes four drugs—isoniazid, rifampicin, pyrazinamide, and ethambutol—for the first 2 months and then isoniazid and rifampicin for the following 4 months.[49]

Once an active case of TB is identified, appropriate drugs of good quality are required in adequate supply for 6 months. It is recommended that fixed-dose combinations of the required drugs be taken daily. Patient adherence with the TB regimen is required for effective therapy. This should be encouraged through a "patient-centered approach" that encourages health education and counseling and consideration of the most appropriate options for drug administration, such as at home, in the community, or in a facility.[50] In 2018, globally, 82% of people diagnosed with drug-susceptible TB were treated successfully and cured of TB.[13]

Treating active drug-susceptible TB through an organized quality-assured care program is highly cost-effective, with fairly recent studies showing the cost ranging from $5 to $50 per DALY averted in most regions. The cost of treating a TB case, in fact, is below $200 in several countries.[13] BCG is cost-effective in reducing severe cases of childhood TB in high-prevalence settings.[48]

The Management of TB/HIV Co-infection

TB is an opportunistic infection of HIV. As the immune system of an HIV-positive person declines, TB is one of the diseases that can develop. This is especially so in populations where many people have latent TB. In addition, TB has been the leading cause of death of adults who are HIV-positive and not on antiretroviral therapy, although cryptococcal meningitis may now be responsible for more deaths of HIV-positive people in Africa than TB.[24]

WHO recommends a number of measures to prevent and manage TB and HIV co-infection, including intensified case finding; giving isoniazid, an antibiotic, to people with HIV to help prevent them from getting TB; and enhancing infection control in healthcare settings.[44] There are still substantial gaps in many countries in managing TB/HIV coinfection in conjunction with these guidelines.[51]

Challenges in TB Prevention and Care

WHO has developed the End TB Strategy, which seeks to end the global TB epidemic by 2035, with a 95% reduction in TB deaths and a drop in incidence to 10 per 100,000 people. It also calls for the elimination of catastrophic costs for TB-affected families. The strategy is based on expanding TB prevention and care through a focus on high-impact interventions in a patient-centered way, working with a wider array of public and private partners, pursuing policy shifts associated with universal health coverage, social protection and poverty alleviation, pursuing basic research, development of new tools, and operational research.[52]

The End TB Strategy also emphasizes the importance of embedding TB care in universal health coverage and further linking TB efforts with the strengthening of health systems. This includes the improvement of laboratory services and infection control and further integrating TB care at the primary level, especially through community-based care. The strategy also highlights the importance of promoting more community-based approaches to information and education about TB as well as the increased involvement of patients, communities, and civil society in TB efforts.[52]

Malaria

The Burden of Malaria

There were 229 million cases of malaria in 2019. By WHO region, approximately 94% of these cases were in Africa, 3% in South-East Asia, and 2% in the Eastern Mediterranean. It is estimated that 409,000 people died of malaria in 2019. Approximately 94% of these deaths were in Africa and 67% were among children under five. Important progress has been made against malaria until recently, with deaths declining from 736,000 to 409,000 from 2000 to 2019.[53] This was largely the result of greater use of insecticide-treated bed nets, indoor residual spraying, and better treatment on the basis of a confirmed diagnosis.

Malaria is caused by parasites in the genus *Plasmodium*, five species of which infect humans: *P. falciparum*, *P. vivax*, *P. ovale*, *P. malariae*, and *P. knowlesi*. These parasite species exist in different proportions in different regions of the world. For example, *P. falciparum* dominates in Africa, *P. vivax* occurs in temperate zones, and *P. ovale* is found in South Asia and tropical Africa.[54] *P. knowlesi* is the least common form and primarily affects macaques. However, it can also infect humans, especially in forested areas of South-East Asia.[55] Malaria is spread by the bite of the female *Anopheles* mosquito.

The most important risk factor for malaria is being bitten by mosquitoes that carry the malaria parasite. This risk varies with the feeding habits of various species of mosquitoes, the climate, and the time of year. Some people have a degree of immunity to malaria from having grown up in malarial zones, and the risks of contracting malaria increase if one does not have such immunity.[55]

Pregnant women who contract malaria are at high risk of giving birth to low-birthweight children. Malaria in pregnancy is also associated with spontaneous abortion, stillbirth, premature delivery, and severe anemia in the mother and the baby.[55] An earlier study suggested that 3 to 15% of African mothers suffered severe anemia, accounting for 10,000 malaria-related anemia deaths per year.[55] It was further estimated that globally, malaria would cause approximately 30% of low birthweight in newborns and between 75,000 and 200,000 infant deaths per year.[56]

The Costs and Consequences of Malaria

The cost of malaria at the family level is substantial because individuals often have malaria up to five times per year. In one study in Ghana, for example, there were 11 cases of malaria per household, per year, on average.[28] These same studies showed that individuals lost 1 to 5 work days per episode of malaria, that the indirect cost of dealing with their illness was greater than the direct costs of treatment, and that each episode of malaria probably cost an adult about 2% of his or her annual income.[28] In many African countries, malaria typically accounts for 30% or more of outpatient visits and hospital admissions for children under five years of age.[57]

Addressing the Burden of Malaria

Treatment of malaria should be initiated within 24 hours based on a confirmed diagnosis.[58] Traditionally, diagnoses were supposed to be made through a microscopic examination of a blood smear, but this was often not done. However, a rapid diagnostic test (RDT) was developed to make it easier to test for malaria in low-resource settings, and the use of these kits has become widespread. Approximately 75% of the malaria tests in 2017 in Africa were RDTs. In addition, an estimated 245 million RDTs were used by national malaria programs in 2017, mostly in Africa.[59]

WHO today recommends artemisinin-based combination therapies for treating uncomplicated malaria caused by *P. falciparum* and for treating *P. vivax* infections that are not responsive to chloroquine.[58] WHO also recommends that pregnant women in areas in Africa where malaria is endemic be treated with intermittent preventive therapy as part of antenatal care.[58] To protect infants in areas of moderate to high transmission of malaria in Africa, WHO recommends that they be given preventive treatment against malaria.[58] In the Sahel region of Africa, with highly seasonal transmission of malaria, WHO recommends that all children under 6 years of age be given seasonal monthly treatment against malaria.[58]

The use of long-lasting insecticide-treated bed nets (ITNs) is another important pillar of malaria control. Bed nets, impregnated with a biologically safe insecticide, are being widely distributed for free and sold by governments, donors, and the private sector. The percentage of people in malaria-endemic areas with access to ITNs increased from 33% in 2010 to 56% in 2017.[57]

Spraying the inside of homes, or indoor residual spraying, is also important. Five insecticides are approved by WHO for indoor residual spraying.[60] Pyrethroids have been the insecticide of choice for spraying, but DDT is also approved for such efforts. Assessments are made to examine resistance to the insecticides and the need to rotate insecticides to slow the development of resistance to them. Particular attention is also being paid to potential environmental risks of the insecticides.[60]

After many years of effort, there has finally been some progress in the development of a malaria vaccine. The RTS,S/ASO1 (RTS,S) vaccine is the first vaccine to provide partial protection against malaria in young children. In clinical trials done among 15,000 children in seven countries in sub-Saharan Africa, the vaccine prevented approximately 40% of cases over four years and about 30% of cases of severe malaria. Who coordinated an effort with Ghana, Kenya, and Malawi to further test the vaccine, which requires four doses.[61] WHO approved the vaccine in October 2021.

Diarrheal Disease
The Burden of Diarrheal Disease

WHO defines diarrhea as "the passage of three or more loose or liquid stools per day (or more frequent passage than is normal for the individual)."[62] Diarrhea is caused by certain bacteria, viruses, and/or parasites that are transmitted by contaminated water or food through the fecal-oral route, such as *Shigella*, *Cholera vibrio*, and rotavirus. Diarrheal disease agents can be spread by dirty utensils, dirty hands, or flies. Poor recognition of the extent of illness, failed home care, and lack of knowledge about simple therapies increase the severity of diarrhea.[63]

Diarrheal diseases most significantly impact the poor, especially children, in low- and middle-income countries. Poor housing, crowding, lack of safe water and sanitation, cohabitation with domestic animals, lack of refrigeration for food storage, and poor personal and community hygiene all contribute to the transmission of diarrheal disease agents. In addition, poor nutrition contributes to poor immunity and increases the frequency and severity of diarrhea. This contributes to a vicious cycle of diarrhea and undernutrition because diarrhea can cause malnutrition. Diarrhea causes severe dehydration and a loss of body water and can kill infants and young children very quickly.[64]

Diarrheal disease mortality has decreased significantly in the past 30 years. This decline has largely been due to improved infant nutrition, better disease recognition by families and healthcare providers, improved care seeking, appropriate use of oral rehydration therapy, increasing rates of coverage of the measles vaccine, and the growing use of the rotavirus vaccine.

Nonetheless, diarrhea remains a major cause of death and sickness for children younger than five years. WHO estimated in 2016 that there were about 1.7 billion cases of diarrheal disease among children and that diarrhea was responsible for 525,000 deaths of such children.[62] WHO also estimated that children under three years of age in low- and middle-income countries suffer on average about three episodes of diarrhea annually, although rates vary worldwide.[62]

Diarrheal diseases are the cause of about 10% of all deaths of children under five globally, about 13% in sub-Saharan Africa, and about 7% in South Asia. Diarrheal diseases are the third leading cause of death for under five children globally and in sub-Saharan Africa, and the fourth leading cause of death for under five children in South Asia, behind neonatal disorders and lower respiratory infections.[1]

Addressing the Burden of Diarrhea

There are several major disease prevention strategies for diarrhea. The first is access to safe water and improved sanitation coupled with better handwashing with soap. Second is the promotion of exclusive breastfeeding for six months. This is advantageous to the child because the child receives both maternal antibodies and a nutritious and uncontaminated meal. Mothers benefit from an increased birth interval and a healthier child. This can be coupled with improved complementary feeding, which can be introduced hygienically with breastfeeding after six months. Good personal and food hygiene is also central to reducing diarrheal disease, which will, hopefully, follow efforts at health education and hygiene promotion. The next measure is rotavirus immunization.[64] Measles immunization is also important to reducing diarrheal disease. Data indicate a clear link between measles immunization and reduced incidence and deaths from diarrhea. Ensuring that an increasing share of children have sufficient levels of vitamin A by raising supplementation rates is also important.[64]

A number of case management interventions can significantly reduce the severity and mortality of diarrheal disease. The use of oral rehydration therapy (ORT) is the most cost-effective case management intervention, especially if homemade solutions are administered. Related to this, it was also estimated that zinc supplementation during an acute diarrhea episode lasting 10 to 14 days could reduce the duration of diarrhea by approximately 25% and stool volume by 30%. Continuing to feed nutrient-rich foods is also important.[64]

Neglected Tropical Diseases
The Burden of Neglected Tropical Diseases

WHO lists 22 neglected tropical diseases (NTDs). Together, these affect more than 1 billion people. Some of the most prevalent of these diseases and the number of people they infect annually are ascariasis (roundworm) — 819 million; hookworm — 439 million; trichuriasis (whipworm) — 465 million; schistosomiasis — 102 million; Lymphatic filariasis — 36 million; onchocerciasis — 21 million; and trachoma — 1.9 million.[65]

NTDs are diseases of poverty, affecting nearly everyone in the "bottom billion" of the world's poorest people. NTDs are especially prevalent in subtropical and tropical climates. Women and children who live in unhygienic environments with limited access to clean water and sanitary methods of waste disposal face the biggest threat of NTDs. Pregnant women also face special risks from some NTDs. People engaged in farming are particularly susceptible to NTDs because of their close contact with soil, which can harbor many of the parasites and worms that cause NTDs. People who live in Africa and rely on rivers for drinking and bathing are also more likely to be affected by certain NTDs, such as onchocerciasis.

Individuals whose labor or domestic chores are centered on freshwater sources are also more likely to contract NTDs.[66] Living in close proximity to livestock and to the vectors of infection increases risk as well.[66]

Moreover, the burden of the worm diseases not only concerns being infected but also the number of worms in the body. Children of preschool age generally have the greatest number of worms. In addition, the prevalence of intestinal worms in many school-aged children in the most heavily burdened countries is exceptionally high.[66]

NTDs can have a terrible impact on health, impede child growth and development, harm pregnant women, and often cause long-term debilitating illnesses. They cause an extraordinary amount of ill health, disability, and disfigurement. Some deaths are also associated with NTDs, especially from schistosomiasis. Those who suffer from NTDs are frequently shunned by their families and their communities. In addition, people with these diseases are often unable to work productively, leading to enormous economic losses for them, their families, and the nations in which they live.

Many diseases kill more people than NTDs do. However, NTDs can make people sick for long periods of time and can cause long-lasting disabilities. In fact, some studies suggest that NTDs result in about half as many DALYs annually as are caused by malaria.[1]

Despite their significance, insufficient financial support was provided until recently to address NTDs, compared with the burden of ill health they cause. This was especially regrettable because significant progress has been made to control or eliminate some of the NTDs, including Chagas disease, lymphatic filariasis, onchocerciasis, Guinea worm, and leprosy. It is also lamentable because a package of drugs to prevent six NTDs is available for about 50 cents per year through mass drug administration.[67]

The Consequences of the Neglected Tropical Diseases

NTDs can have debilitating social and economic consequences as well as a major impact on the health and well-being of those infected. On the clinical side, for example, trachoma can lead to redness and swelling of the eye, sensitivity to light, corneal scarring, and eventually permanent blindness. Schistosomiasis is associated with painful and/or bloody urination, bloody diarrhea, enlargement of the liver and/or spleen, and liver cancer; it is also the deadliest of the NTDs. Lymphatic filariasis is well known for the remarkable swelling it can cause in the limbs and genitals. Onchocerciasis leads to skin problems and blindness.

The helminthic infections are generally associated with abdominal pain, loss of appetite, malnutrition, diarrhea, and anemia. In addition, chronic helminthic infection in children can limit their physical and mental development. Pregnant women with hookworm are at high risk of giving birth to low-birthweight babies, of birthing babies who fail to thrive, and of having poor milk production. In addition, pregnant women with anemia, commonly caused by hookworm in low-income countries, are three and a half times more likely to die during childbirth than women who are not anemic. This risk is especially significant because one-quarter to one-third of pregnant women in sub-Saharan Africa are infected with hookworm.[68] Whipworm also can lead to severe growth restriction in children.

Social stigma is a major consequence of the NTDs. Many of the NTDs cause disability and disfigurement, resulting in individuals being shunned by their families and their communities. When not treated, for example, leprosy can cause terrible skin lesions that have been stigmatized since biblical times. Few health conditions are as stigmatizing as the swelling of limbs and genitalia that can result from lymphatic filariasis. Individuals who are stigmatized are less likely to seek diagnosis and treatment. Social stigma is particularly demoralizing for young women because they are often left unmarried and unable to work in settings where the social value of a woman has much to do with her marital status.

NTDs also have a major impact on the productivity of individuals and the economic prospects of communities and nations. Children are disproportionately affected by NTDs and often suffer long-term consequences from them. In some areas, hookworm infection in school-age children contributes to a drop in school attendance by over 20%, and poor school attendance and poor school performance reduce future earnings. In fact, hookworm has been shown to reduce future wage-earning capacity in some affected areas by up to 43%.[68]

NTDs adversely affect economic productivity at the individual, family, community, and national levels. NTDs lead to important losses in income that cause some families to sell assets to try to stay financially solvent. In addition, regions severely affected by onchocerciasis often cannot be used effectively for economic activities such as farming because families that try to live in these areas are at risk of being blinded by the disease. WHO estimates that blindness due to trachoma costs the world between $2.9 and $5.3 billion annually.[69]

Addressing the Neglected Tropical Diseases

There has been considerable progress in the fight against a number of NTDs, including continuing declines in the incidence of the diseases discussed, as well as a growing number of people treated for them. The following are other examples of progress: Guinea worm has been nearly eradicated; Morocco and Oman have eliminated trachoma; six countries have eliminated lymphatic filariasis and a further 18 countries no longer require mass drug administration for this disease; and onchocerciasis has been nearly eliminated in the Americas.[66]

The successes against NTDs thus far suggest that additional progress can be made rapidly and at relatively low cost to combat the exceptional number of cases of NTDs that remain worldwide. However, further progress is likely to require concerted action in a number of areas, including scaling up the treatment package, focusing on deworming, integrating NTD control with other programs and universal health coverage, and developing new technologies to address NTD control.

Following the lessons of the onchocerciasis program and others, this package can be implemented rapidly with the help of medicine distributors who are chosen from among members of the affected communities through community-directed treatment.[70] This type of community-directed treatment for onchocerciasis with ivermectin has proven particularly successful in rural Africa.[70]

Periodic deworming of young children is also a best buy in global health and should be a major focus of attention.[71] Deworming is the single most cost-effective means to improve school attendance. There is also historical evidence that deworming improves children's cognitive skills and their potential to learn, which leads to greater literacy and higher productivity among adults.[72] In addition, recent studies have shown that deworming children may significantly reduce the burden of malaria because children infected with ascariasis are twice as likely to get severe malaria as children who are not infected.[68]

At the same time as countries seek to prevent and treat NTDs broadly through programs of mass drug administration or treatment of specific diseases, they need to work with communities to address the underlying risks for NTDs. For the NTDs discussed here, these risks overwhelmingly relate to the unsanitary living conditions of the poor. It will remain important for people to better understand the importance of good hygiene, to have better access to safe water and sanitary disposal of human waste, and to eliminate worm and parasite breeding sites. In the long run, progress in all of these directions will help to reduce the burden of NTDs and sustain such reductions. Unfortunately, however, these developments are not likely to take place quickly. The fastest and most cost-effective route to reducing the burden of NTDs will be to implement the package of prevention and treatment discussed in this chapter as quickly as possible.

Discussion Questions

1. What is the relative importance of communicable diseases to deaths and DALYs in different country income groups?
2. How can the world prepare better for the next pandemic than it did for the 2019 novel coronavirus?
3. What are some of the most important factors contributing to the development of drug resistance?
4. Who is most affected by TB and why?
5. What role could treatment play in trying to reduce the burden of HIV/AIDS?

References

1. IHME. *GBD Compare Viz Hub*. nd. Retrieved from: https://vizhub.healthdata.org/gbd-compare/
2. Fauci AS. Robert H. Ebert memorial lecture. Emerging and re-emerging infectious diseases: the perpetual challenge. New York, NY: Milbank Memorial Fund; 2005.
3. Heymann DL. Emerging and re-emerging infectious diseases from plague and cholera to Ebola and AIDS: a potential for international spread that transcends the defenses of any single country. *J Contin Crisis Manag*. 2005;13(1):29–31.
4. Heymann D. Emerging and re-emerging infections. In: W. Kirch, ed. *Encyclopedia of Public Health*. New York, NY: Springer; 2008.
5. Jones KE, Patel NG, Levy MA, et al. Global trends in emerging infectious diseases. *Nature*. 2008;451(7181):990–993.
6. World Health Organization. *Global Tuberculosis Report 2019*. 2019A. Retrieved from https://www.who.int/tb/publications/factsheet_global.pdf?ua=1
7. National Institutes of Health. *Microbial evolution and co-adaptation: a tribute to the life and scientific legacies of Joshua Lederberg. Workshop summary*. Institute of Medicine Forum on Microbial Threats. Washington, DC: National Academies Press; 2009.
8. Nugent R, Beck E, Beith A. *The race against drug resistance*. Washington, DC: Center for Global Development; 2010.

9. Okeke IN, Laxminarayan R, Bhutta ZA, et al. Antimicrobial resistance in developing countries. Part I: recent trends and current status. *Lancet Infect Dis.* 2005A;5(8):481–493.

10. Okeke IN, Klugman KP, Bhutta ZA, et al. Antimicrobial resistance in developing countries. Part II: strategies for containment. *Lancet Infect Dis.* 2005B;5(9):568–580.

11. Laxminarayan R, Bhutta ZA, Duse A, et al. Drug resistance. In: Jamison DT, Breman JG, Measham AR, et al., eds. *Disease control priorities in developing countries.* 2nd ed. New York, NY: Oxford University Press; 2006:1031–1051.

12. Heymann DL. The microbial threat in fragile times: Balancing known and unknown risks. *Bulletin of the World Health Organization.* 2002;80(3):179.

13. World Health Organization (WHO). *Global tuberculosis report 2018.* Geneva, Switzerland; 2018A.

14. World Health Organization. *International health regulations.* 2nd ed. Geneva, Switzerland; 2005.

15. Global Health Security Agenda. *About.* nd. Retrieved from https://www.ghsagenda.org/

16. World Health Organization (WHO). *Global action plan on antimicrobial resistance.* Geneva, Switzerland; 2015A.

17. World Health Organization (WHO). *WHO report on surveillance of antibiotic consumption: 2016–2018 early implementation.* Geneva, Switzerland; 2018B.

18. Tacconelli E, Carrara E, Savoldi A, et al. Discovery, research, and development of new antibiotics: the WHO priority list of antibiotic-resistant bacteria and tuberculosis. *Lancet Infect Dis.* 2018;18(3):318–327.

19. World Economic Forum. *Outbreak readiness and business impact protecting lives and livelihoods across the global economy.* Geneva, Switzerland: 2019.

20. Quick JD, Fryer B. *The end of pandemics: the looming threat to humanity and how to stop it.* New York, NY: St. Martin's Press; 2019.

21. Gostin LO, Katz R. The international health regulations: the governing framework for global health security. *The Milbank Quarterly.* 2016;94(2):264–313.

22. UNAIDS. *Global HIV & AIDS Statistics – 2020 Fact Sheet.* nd. Retrieved February 11, 2021, from https://www.unaids.org/en/resources/fact-sheet#:~:text=GLOBAL%20HIV%20STATISTICS&text=1.7%20million%20%5B1.2%20million%E2%80%932.2,the%20epidemic%20(end%202019).

23. Centers for Disease Control and Prevention. *Estimated per act risk of acquisition of HIV. MMWR.* 2005;54(RR02):1–20.

24. Avert. Cryptococcal meningitis remains a leading killer of people living with HIV. 2017. Retrieved from: https://www.avert.org/news/cryptococcal-meningitis-remains-leading-killer-people-living-hiv

25. World Health Organization. *Latest HIV estimates and updates on HIV policies uptake, November 2020.* 2020A. Retrieved from: https://www.who.int/docs/default-source/hiv-hq/latest-hiv-estimates-and-updates-on-hiv-policies-uptake-november2020.pdf?sfvrsn=10a0043d_12

26. UNAIDS. *Global HIV & AIDS Statistics – 2020 Fact Sheet.* nd. Retrieved February 11, 2021 from https://www.unaids.org/en/resources/fact-sheet#:~:text=GLOBAL%20HIV%20STATISTICS&text=1.7%20million%20%5B1.2%20million%E2%80%932.2,the%20epidemic%20(end%202019)

27. UNAIDS. *Fast track: Ending the AIDS epidemic by 2030.* Geneva, Switzerland; 2014.

28. Russell S. The economic burden of illness for households in developing countries: a review of studies focusing on malaria, tuberculosis, and human immunodeficiency virus/acquired immunodeficiency syndrome. *Am J Trop Med Hyg.* 2004;71(2 suppl):147–155.

29. Unicef. HIV statistics—global and regional trends. 2020. Retrieved February 12, 2021, from https://data.unicef.org/topic/hivaids/global-regional-trends/

30. MSF Treatment Access Campaign. *Stopping senseless deaths.* 2018. Retrieved from https://www.msf.org/sites/msf.org/files/2018-08/HIV_Brief_Stopping_Senseless_Deaths_ENG_2018.pdf

31. Resch S, Ryckman T, Hecht R. Funding AIDS programmes in the era of shared responsibility: an analysis of domestic spending in 12 low-income and middle-income countries. *Lancet Glob Health.* 2015;3(1):e52–e61.

32. Pio P, Seck AM. International response to the HIV/AIDS epidemic: planning for success. *Bull World Health Org.* 2001;79 (12).

33. Kurth AE, Celum C, Baeten JM, Vermund SH, Wasserheit JN. Combination HIV prevention: significance, challenges, and opportunities. *Current HIV/AIDS Reports*, 2011;8(1):62–72. doi: 10.1007/s11904-010-0063-3

34. Avert. Prevention of Mother-To-Child Transmission (PMTCT) of HIV. nd. Retrieved from https://www.avert.org/professionals/hiv-programming/prevention/prevention-mother-child

35. World Health Organization (WHO). *Guidelines on HIV and infant feeding 2010.* Geneva, Switzerland; 2010A.

36. Centers for Disease Control and Prevention (CDC). *Male circumcision and risk for HIV transmission: Implications for the United States.* 2008. Retrieved from http://stacks.cdc.gov /view/cdc/13545/

37. Dickson KE, Tran NT, Samuelson JL, et al. Voluntary medical male circumcision: a framework analysis of policy and program implementation in Eastern and Southern Africa. *PLOS Med.* 2011;8(11):e1001133. doi: 10.1371/journal.pmed.1001133

38. World Health Organization. *Global tuberculosis report 2020.* Geneva: World Health Organization; 2020B. Retrieved from https://www.who.int/teams/global-tuberculosis-programme/tb -reports

39. World Health Organization (WHO). *Tuberculosis: key facts.* 2018C. Retrieved from https://www .who.int/en/news-room/fact-sheets/detail/tuberculosis

40. Centers for Disease Control and Prevention (CDC). *Basic TB facts.* 2015. Retrieved from http:// www.cdc.gov/tb/topic/basics/

41. World Health Organization (WHO), World Organization for Animal Health (OIE), Food and Agriculture Organization of the United Nations (FAO), & International Union Against Tuberculosis and Lung Disease. *Zoonotic tuberculosis.* 2017. Retrieved from https://www.who .int/tb/areas-of-work/zoonotic-tb/ZoonoticTBfactsheet2017.pdf?ua=1

42. Centers for Disease Control and Prevention (CDC). *Tuberculosis: TB risk factors.* nd, B. Retrieved from http://www.cdc.gov/tb/topic/basics/risk.htm

43. World Health Organization (WHO). *Tuberculosis diagnostics: automated real-time DNA amplification test for rapid and simultaneous detection of TB and rifampicin resistance: Xpert MTB/RIF assay.* nd, B. Retrieved from https://www.who.int/tb/publications/factsheet_xpert .pdf?ua=1

44. World Health Organization (WHO). *Global tuberculosis report 2014.* Geneva, Switzerland: 2014A.

45. World Health Organization. *Tuberculosis. Drug resistant tuberculosis.* nd, C. Retrieved from https://www.who.int/tb/areas-of-work/drug-resistant-tb/en/

46. World Health Organization (WHO). *Gender, equity, and human rights. Gender and tuberculosis.* nd, D. Retrieved from https://www.who.int/gender-equity-rights/knowledge/a85584/en/

47. Chand N, Singh T, Khalsa JS, Verma V, Rathore JS. A study of socio-economic impact of tuberculosis on patients and their family. *Chest.* 2004;126(4):832S.

48. Dye C, Floyd K. Tuberculosis. In: Jamison DT, Breman JG, Measham AR, et al., eds. *Disease control priorities in developing countries.* 2nd ed. New York, NY: Oxford University Press; 2006:289–312.

49. World Health Organization (WHO). *Guidelines for the treatment of tuberculosis* 4th ed. 2010. Geneva, Switzerland. Retrieved from: http://apps.who.int/iris/bitstream/handle/10665 /44165/9789241547833_eng.pdf;jsessionid=E14218163B65E53D16D17784008401E5? sequence=1

50. World Health Organization (WHO). *WHO guidelines for treatment of drug-susceptible TB and patient care.* 2017A. Retrieved from https://www.who.int/tb/publications/2017/DS_TB _treatmentFactsheet.pdf?ua=1

51. World Health Organization (WHO). *HIV-associated tuberculosis.* 2018D. Retrieved from https:// www.who.int/tb/areas-of-work/tb-hiv/tbhiv_factsheet.pdf?ua=1

52. World Health Organization (WHO). *The end TB strategy.* Geneva, Switzerland; 2014B.

53. World Health Organization. *World Malaria Report 2020: 20 years of global progress and challenges.* 2020C. Geneva: World Health Organization. Retrieved from https://www.who.int /publications/i/item/9789240015791

54. CDC. (nd). Malaria. Frequently Asked Questions (FAQs). Retrieved from https://www.cdc.gov /malaria/about/faqs.html

55. Breman JG, Mills A, Snow RW, Mulligan JA. Conquering malaria. In: Jamison DT, Breman JG, Measham AR, et al., eds. *Disease Control Priorities in Developing Countries.* 2nd ed. New York, NY: Oxford University Press; 2006:413–432.

56. World Health Organization (WHO). *Malaria in pregnant women.* 2017B. Retrieved from http:// www.who.int/malaria/areas/high_risk_groups/pregnancy/en/

57. World Health Organization (WHO). *10 facts on malaria.* 2016. Retrieved from https://www .who.int/features/factfiles/malaria/en

58. World Health Organization (WHO). *Malaria: overview of malaria treatment.* 2018F. Retrieved from https://www.who.int/malaria/areas/treatment/overview/en/

59. World Health Organization (WHO). *World malaria report 2018.* Geneva, Switzerland; 2018F.

60. President's Malaria Initiative. *Indoor residual spraying.* nd. Retrieved from http://www.pmi.gov /how-we-work/technical-areas/indoor-residual-spraying

61. World Health Organization (WHO). *Q and A on the malaria vaccine implementation program (MVIP).* 2019. Retrieved from https://www.who.int/malaria/media/malaria-vaccine-implementation -qa/en/

62. World Health Organization (WHO). *Diarrhoeal disease: Key facts.* 2017C. Retrieved from https://www.who.int/news-room/fact-sheets/detail/diarrhoeal-disease

63. Keusch GT, Fontaine O, Bhargava A, Boschi-Pinto C. Diarrheal diseases. In: Jamison DT, Breman JG, Measham AR, et al., eds. *Disease Control Priorities in Developing Countries.* 2nd ed. New York, NY: Oxford University Press;2006:371–388.

64. UNICEF & World Health Organization. *Diarrhoea: Why children are still dying and what can be done.* New York, NY; 2009.

65. Kaiser Family Foundation. The U.S. government and global neglected tropical disease efforts. 2020. Retrieved February 12, 2021 from https://www.kff.org/global-health-policy/fact-sheet /the-u-s-government-and-global-neglected-tropical-diseases/

66. World Health Organization (WHO). *Neglected tropical diseases: implementing the WHO roadmap on neglected tropical diseases—partners celebrate five years of collaboration.* 2017E. Retrieved from https://www.who.int/neglected_diseases/news/WHO_Roadmap_five_years_of _collaboration/en/

67. Centers for Disease Control and Prevention (CDC). *Neglected tropical diseases.* nd, C. Retrieved from https://www.cdc.gov/globalhealth/ntd/diseases/index.html

68. Hotez P. Hookworm and poverty. *Ann New York Acad Sci.* 2008;1136(1):38–44.

69. World Health Organization. *Trachoma.* 2018G. Retrieved from https://www.who.int/en/news -room/fact-sheets/detail/trachoma

70. World Health Organization (WHO). *Onchocerciasis.* 2018. Retrieved from https://www .who.int/news-room/fact-sheets/detail/onchocerciasisWorld Health Organization (WHO). *Onchocerciasis.* 2018. Retrieved from https://www.who.int/news-room/fact-sheets/detail /onchocerciasis

71. Copenhagen Consensus Center. Homepage. nd. Retrieved from http://www.copenhagen consensus.com/Home.aspx

72. Evidence Action. *Deworm the world initiative: the evidence for deworming.* nd. Retrieved from http://www.evidenceaction.org/dewormtheworld/

CHAPTER 7

Noncommunicable Diseases, Mental Disorders, and Injuries

LEARNING OBJECTIVES

By the end of this chapter, the reader will be able to do the following:

- Describe the burden of noncommunicable diseases and mental disorders worldwide
- Discuss the most important risk factors for the burden of these conditions
- Outline the costs and consequences of selected noncommunicable diseases and mental disorders
- Review measures that can be taken to address the burden of these conditions in cost-effective and fair ways

VIGNETTES

Roberto was 45 years old and lived in Bogota, Colombia. He had a government desk job and had been overweight for most of his adult life. He got little exercise. He had read about increasing rates of diabetes in Colombia but still thought this was largely a disease of people in rich countries. Last year, Roberto started feeling thirsty all of the time, had dry mouth, and felt weak after exertion. He went to his doctor and was diagnosed with type 2 diabetes.

Lai Ying was a factory worker who lived in Guangdong Province, China. Until recently, she had been a happy and healthy young woman. Lately, however, Lai Ying had felt very unhappy, did not feel like getting out of bed in the morning, did not want to go to work, and had no energy when she was at work. Lai Ying's family noticed that she was not eating properly and that she was not herself. However, they thought she was having a difficult time at work or with a boyfriend and that she would soon be fine. After some months of this behavior, Lai Ying consumed an overdose of sleeping pills and died by suicide.

Key Definitions

In this text, we shall consistently use the term **noncommunicable disease**. This will include all causes that are included in the Global Burden of Disease Study 2019 under the category of noncommunicable diseases, including mental disorders.[1]

This chapter will focus on selected noncommunicable diseases. This includes cancers, cardiovascular disease, chronic obstructive pulmonary disease, vision and hearing loss, and mental health disorders. Including mental disorders in the chapter title is intended to signal the coverage of the chapter and the importance of mental health.

The Importance of Noncommunicable Diseases

Noncommunicable diseases are of immense importance worldwide. The burden of these conditions is greater than the burden of communicable diseases in low- and middle-income countries as well as in high-income countries. Only in sub-Saharan Africa is the burden of communicable diseases higher than that of noncommunicable diseases.[2]

Moreover, the burden of noncommunicable diseases will increase in low- and middle-income countries as they develop economically, become more integrated with the global economy, urbanize, and age. Among the most important of the noncommunicable health conditions that low- and middle-income countries face are **ischemic heart disease**, **stroke**, **chronic obstructive pulmonary disease (COPD)**, **diabetes**, cancers, musculoskeletal disorders, and mental health disorders.[2]

The risk factors for several noncommunicable diseases relate to lifestyle, much of which is **modifiable**. By engaging in appropriate health behaviors, it is possible for most people to considerably reduce the risk of getting heart disease, stroke, COPD, some cancers, or diabetes.

The Burden of Noncommunicable Diseases

Cardiovascular Disease (CVD)

Ischemic heart disease was the leading specific cause of death globally for all age groups and both sexes in 2019, causing 16% of all deaths, followed by stroke, which was responsible for approximately 12% of all deaths.[2]

Ischemic heart disease is the fifth leading cause of death in low-income countries. However, it is the leading cause of death for both sexes and all ages in lower middle-, upper middle-, and high-income countries. Stroke is the second leading cause of death in lower middle-, upper middle-, and high-income countries, but is the fourth leading cause in low-income countries.[2]

Ischemic heart disease was the second leading cause of disability-adjusted life years (DALYs) and stroke was the third leading cause of DALYs globally among all age groups and both sexes in 2019. For low-income countries, ischemic heart disease was the tenth leading cause of DALYs, and stroke was the eighth leading cause of DALYs. In the lower middle-income countries, ischemic heart disease was the second leading cause and stroke was the fourth. In the upper middle-income countries, ischemic heart disease was the leading cause and stroke was second. In the high-income countries, ischemic heart disease was the leading cause of DALYs and stroke was the third leading cause.[2]

Given the limited access to prevention programs or appropriate treatment, deaths from CVD generally occur earlier in life in low- and middle-income countries than in high-income countries. In India, for example, approximately 50% of the CVD deaths occur in people under 70, compared with only 22% in high-income countries.[3]

Men have a higher risk of heart disease than women who are premenopausal, but postmenopausal women have the same risk of cardiovascular disease as men. In addition, men and women have similar risks of stroke. The medical history of one's family is also significant. If a male relative had coronary heart disease before 55 years of age or a female relative before 65 years of age, he has a higher risk of heart disease. Ancestry is also relevant, as people of African or Asian descent have higher risks than other groups. Aging also increases risk, with the risk of a stroke doubling every 10 years after age 55.[4]

Some of the modifiable risk factors for cardiovascular disease include hypertension, which is the biggest risk factor for stroke, and a major risk factor for heart disease. Tobacco use is also a major risk factor for CVD, with higher risks for women and those who started smoking early and smoke a lot. High levels of cholesterol, which are linked to a diet high in saturated fats and lack of physical activity, are also risks. The lack of physical activity is a risk for obesity that in turn is a risk for diabetes, which doubles one's risk of CVD. Excess alcohol consumption is also associated with heart disease.[4]

Social factors can be important risks for CVD. There is good evidence that higher risks of CVD are associated, for example, with poverty, stress, and being isolated socially. Depression is also an important risk factor for CVD.[4]

Diabetes

There are several types of diabetes. The two most common are called type 1 and type 2 diabetes. Type 1 diabetes is thought to be an autoimmune disorder that attacks and destroys the cells in the pancreas that produce insulin. Without insulin, the body is not able to use glucose (blood sugar) for energy. To treat the disease, a person must inject insulin, follow a diet plan, exercise daily, and test blood sugar several times a day.[5] Type 1 diabetes usually begins before the age of 30. Type 2 diabetes is the most common form of diabetes mellitus, present in about 90 to 95% of all people with diabetes. People with type 2 diabetes are able to produce insulin; however, they either do not make enough insulin or their bodies do not efficiently use the insulin that they do make.[5]

There is also a third type of diabetes, generally referred to as **gestational diabetes**. A high blood glucose level—hyperglycemia—that is diagnosed first in pregnancy is referred to as **hyperglycemia in pregnancy** or

gestational diabetes mellitus (GDM). The International Diabetes Federation (IDF) estimates that approximately 16% of pregnancies are associated with GDM.[6]

IDF estimated that 463 million people aged 20 to 79 years had diabetes in 2019, which was 9.3% of that population globally.[7,8] IDF also estimates that there were 1.1 million children and adolescents aged 0 to 19 years in the world who suffered from type 1 diabetes in 2019 and 4.2 million deaths from diabetes that year. IDF estimates that almost 80% of the people with diabetes lived in low- or middle-income countries[8] and that the prevalence of diabetes is 4% in low-income countries, 9.5% in middle-income countries, and 10.4% in high-income countries. The highest rates of prevalence are found in some Pacific islands, where approximately 30% of the population has diabetes. The Global Burden of Disease Study estimated that diabetes was the eighth leading cause of death worldwide in 2019 among all age groups and both sexes.[2] IDF also estimates that 700 million adults will have diabetes by 2045.[7]

Diabetes has a number of important and costly complications. Among the most common are eye problems that can cause blindness, kidney problems, circulatory problems that can result in amputation of the lower extremities, stroke, and coronary heart disease. About two-thirds of people with diabetes have some disability, compared with less than one-third of people without diabetes.[9]

The risk factors for type 1 diabetes are still being studied. However, type 1 diabetes is associated with a family history of diabetes. In addition, environmental factors, increased weight and height development, increased maternal age at birth, and exposure to some viral infections have been linked to developing type 1 diabetes.[10] Type 2 diabetes is also associated with a family history of diabetes. In addition, it is associated with diet and physical inactivity, obesity, insulin resistance, ancestry, and increasing age.[10,11] In high-income countries, less-educated and lower-income individuals have higher rates of diabetes than better-educated and wealthier people.[12]

Chronic Obstructive Pulmonary Disease (COPD)

COPD refers to chronic lung diseases that cause limitations in lung airflow. The most common symptoms are shortness of breath, excessive sputum production, and a chronic cough. COPD is a life-threatening disease; it can progress to death.[13]

The main risk factors for COPD are tobacco smoking; household air pollution; ambient particulate matter pollution; occupational exposures to dust, chemicals, fumes, and other irritants; and frequent lower respiratory infections as a child.[13,14] Exposure to household air pollution as a child can also be a risk factor for developing COPD later in life.[14] COPD cannot be cured. However, treatments can alleviate symptoms, reduce disability, and prolong life.

Males and females now have roughly equal risk of being affected by COPD.[13] In 2019, COPD was the third leading cause of death globally and the sixth leading cause of DALYs globally. COPD was the 10th leading cause of death in low-income countries and the third leading cause in lower and upper middle-income countries. It was the fifth leading cause of death in high-income countries.[2]

Cancer

All forms of cancer were associated with almost 18% of all deaths in 2019 and combined were the second leading cause of death globally after cardiovascular disease. All forms of cancer combined led to more deaths than either ischemic heart disease or stroke when considered separately.[2] Approximately 70% of all cancer deaths occur in low- and middle-income countries.[15]

Globally, all forms of cancer contributed to almost 10% of all DALYs in 2019. This was the second leading cause of DALYs after CVD. However, as with deaths, all forms of cancer when taken together led to more DALYs than either ischemic heart disease or stroke.[2]

WHO has estimated that among the most commonly occurring cancers worldwide are lung, breast, colorectal, prostate, skin, and stomach cancers.[16] The cancers that cause the most death are lung, colorectal, stomach, liver, and breast cancers. The prevalence of different cancers varies by region: liver cancers are uniquely important in Africa. Cervical cancer is a much larger share of all cancers in Africa than elsewhere. Stomach cancers are uniquely important in the WHO Western Pacific region. Bladder cancers are a larger share of the total cancers in Europe.[16]

Incidence rates remain highest in higher-income regions due to longer average life spans, but mortality is relatively much higher in lower and middle-income countries, likely due to a lack of early detection and lack of access to treatment facilities.[16] Moreover, many low- and middle-income countries face a double burden of cancer due to cancers caused by infectious agents combined with cancers associated with behavioral risks. Decreasing mortality trends in high-income countries can largely be attributed to decreases in risk factors, such as changing smoking habits, especially in men, plus better screening and early detection and improved treatment.[17]

There are many risk factors for cancer, and they vary by the type of cancer. Tobacco use is one of the greatest risk factors for cancer in general. Tobacco is most directly linked to lung cancer, but using tobacco can also indirectly increase the risk of other cancers, such as prostate and breast cancers. Alcohol is associated with liver, upper digestive tract, breast, and colorectal cancers, whereas diets high in red and processed meats and low in fiber have been associated with colorectal cancer. Obesity is a risk factor for breast (postmenopausal), colorectal, endometrial, kidney, esophageal, and pancreatic cancers. Similarly, low physical activity can be a major risk factor for colon, breast, and endometrial cancers.[18]

As noted, other cancers are associated with infectious agents. Liver cancer, for example, is associated with the hepatitis B virus, cervical cancer is associated with the human papillomavirus (HPV), and stomach cancer is associated with the bacteria *Helicobacter pylori*. Liver cancer is also associated with schistosomiasis, a parasitic worm that is also called "bilharzia," which infects more than 200 million people worldwide.[19] There are also numerous environmental and occupational carcinogens, such as asbestos.

Mental Disorders

The World Health Organization defines **mental health** as "a state of well-being in which every individual realizes his or her own potential, can cope with the normal stresses of life, can work productively and fruitfully, and is able to make a contribution to her or his community."[20]

Four mental disorders contribute the largest share to the burden of mental disorders: **depression**, **schizophrenia**, **anxiety disorders**, and **bipolar affective disorder**.[2]

Mental disorders have generally been thought to be associated overwhelmingly with disability rather than with deaths. However, one reputable, even if dated, study estimated that in 2010, more than 2.2 million deaths may have been associated with depression, 1.3 million with bipolar disorder, and about 110,000 with autism spectrum disorder.[21]

The Global Burden of Disease Study 2019 suggests that mental disorders contributed 4.9% of the total DALYs globally.[2] This is more, for example, than the DALYs associated with unintentional injuries, chronic respiratory diseases, or HIV and sexually transmitted diseases. The study also suggests that there is a significant difference between the burden of mental disorders in females and males. Globally, they are associated with 5.7% of DALYs for females and 4.2% for males. Mental disorders are the largest cause of DALYs for the 15 to 49-year-old age group globally. Mental disorders (including suicide) take a particular toll on older adolescents aged 15 to 19 years. Major depressive disorders are the 4th leading cause of DALYs in this age group and anxiety disorders are the 7th leading cause of DALYs in this age group globally for both sexes.[2] The large disability burden of these conditions is related to the substantial number of people who suffer from mental disorders and the fact that mental disorders often start at relatively young ages, go on for a long time, and are often not cured.

The determinants of mental disorders are complex, not very well understood, and appear to be both genetic and nongenetic. A *Lancet* Commission on Global Mental Health and Sustainable Development suggests that the causes of mental disorders relate to "the complex interplay of psychosocial, environmental, biological, and genetic factors across the life course, but in particular during the sensitive developmental periods of childhood and adolescence."[22] Studies have also suggested that a number of social determinants have an especially important impact on mental health: demographic factors: age, gender, and ethnicity; socioeconomic status: low income, unemployment, income inequality, low education, and low social support; neighborhood factors: inadequate housing, overcrowding, neighborhood violence; environmental events: natural disasters, war, conflict, climate change, and migration; and social change associated with changes in income, urbanization, and environmental degradation.[21]

It is also clear that there is a "vicious cycle" between social determinants and mental disorders because having a mental disorder can cause disability, constrain one's ability to function and earn income, and further immiserate the affected person.[21]

Vision and Hearing Loss

Vision Loss

WHO estimates that about 1 billion people suffer from a vision impairment that could have been prevented or is yet to be addressed. These include more than 200 million people who have moderate or severe distance vision impairment or blindness due to: refractive error, cataract, glaucoma corneal opacities, diabetic retinopathy, and trachoma.[23]

Blindness can also be caused by, among other things, glaucoma, vitamin A deficiency, and rubella. Some blindness also has parasitic and infectious causes, such as trachoma and onchocerciasis, although the number of people who are blind because of these causes has declined as progress has been made against these diseases.[24] Diabetes-related eye disease can also cause blindness. Over 80% of vision loss can be prevented or cured.[25]

The main risk factors for visual impairment are poverty, gender, age, and a lack of access to health services. Cigarette smoking is also a risk factor for cataracts and glaucoma.[26] The causes of vision loss and blindness vary by age and country income group. In young children, the leading cause of blindness in low-income countries is congenital cataracts, whereas in high-income countries, it is eye problems associated with prematurity. In adults in low-income countries, a substantial burden of vision loss and blindness is associated with conditions that could be treated but are not, such as refractive errors and cataracts. In high-income countries, adult vision loss is much more often associated with macular degeneration.[25]

Females are more likely than males to suffer blindness and visual impairment from diabetic retinopathy and cataracts. Males are more likely to suffer visual impairment and blindness due to glaucoma and corneal opacity than females.[27] The Global Burden of Disease Study 2019 suggests that visual impairment and blindness were responsible for about 0.6% of all DALYs in 2019 for both sexes and all ages.[2]

Hearing Loss

WHO estimates that about 432 million adults and 34 million children worldwide have disabling hearing loss.[28] Approximately 80% of them have adult-onset hearing loss and about 20% have childhood-onset hearing loss.[29] About one-third of people over 65 years of age are affected by disabling hearing loss.[29] More males have suffered hearing loss than females, probably as a result of exposure to noise.[29] The 2019 Global Burden of Disease Study indicated that 1.6% of DALYs globally, for all ages and both sexes, could be attributed to hearing loss.[2]

Childhood-onset hearing loss is primarily related to congenital conditions, infection of the ear, or complications of other diseases, such as meningitis. Adult-onset hearing loss is largely related to exposure to noise and chemicals as well as to aging. Poverty, poor hygiene, a failure to get vaccinated, and other causes that contribute to children getting infections are also risk factors for hearing loss.[26] Some medicines and recreational exposures can also cause hearing loss.[28] Population aging will increase the burden of hearing loss.

Tobacco Use

Tobacco is also the second leading risk factor for death in high-income countries, the second in upper middle-income countries, the fourth in lower middle-income countries, and the seventh in low-income countries. Tobacco is the second leading risk factor globally for deaths and the third leading for DALYs.[2]

Ultimately, one-half to two-thirds of those who smoke will die of causes related to tobacco.[30] In addition, half of all tobacco-related deaths occur among people ages 35 to 69.[30] The most common tobacco-related deaths are from CVD; diseases of the respiratory system, such as emphysema; and cancers. Tobacco use can also increase the risk of getting tuberculosis (TB) or dying from it, as well as substantially increase the risk of developing diabetes.[31]

Most tobacco is used through smoking either cigarettes or *bidis*, which are hand-rolled cigarettes used largely in South Asia. It is estimated that about 1.1 billion people smoke worldwide.[32] In all regions of the world, men smoke more than women do. The higher the socioeconomic status and the higher the level of education, the less likely a person is to smoke. Most people who smoke start when they are teenagers. In addition, it is important to note that tobacco is physically addictive and that once one starts to smoke, it is difficult to stop.[33]

Alcohol

Alcohol is a major public health problem. Alcohol use is the tenth leading risk factor for deaths globally and the eighth leading risk factor for DALYs. The importance of alcohol use as a risk factor is greater for males than females and is greater in some regions, such as Europe and Central Asia, than in others.[2]

High-risk drinking increases the risks for hypertension, liver damage, pancreatic damage, hormonal problems, and heart disease.[34] In addition, alcohol intoxication is associated with accidents; injuries; accidental death; and a variety of social problems, including the first sexual encounters of teenagers, unprotected sex, and intimate partner violence. It is also possible to become dependent on alcohol, which has a number of negative psychological and physical consequences. Moreover, fetal alcohol syndrome is associated with low birthweight babies who are at risk of developmental disabilities.

There is very little evidence on the determinants of high-risk drinking, especially in low-income settings. Studies done in high-income countries suggest that lower socioeconomic status and lower educational attainment are risk factors for drinking to the level of intoxication.[34]

The Costs and Consequences of Noncommunicable Diseases, Mental Health Disorders, Tobacco Use, and Alcohol Use

Overview

The economic costs of noncommunicable diseases and mental disorders are substantial and are growing, given the increasing burden of cardiovascular disease and diabetes as well as a number of other conditions, such as vision and hearing loss.

The World Economic Forum commissioned a study in 2011 on noncommunicable diseases in low- and middle-income countries. That study concluded that the cumulative output lost due to these conditions in low- and middle-income countries over the next 2 decades would be $47 trillion. The study also suggested that low- and middle-income countries would bear an increasing share of the costs of these diseases in the future.[35] Another study done recently suggested that, especially for populations without insurance, as many as 60% of the families affected by NCDs faced catastrophic, out-of-pocket healthcare expenditures.[36] WHO has also estimated that implementing a package of "best buys" to address NCDs, which is discussed later, could generate $350 billion in additional economic activity between 2018 and 2030.[37]

The International Diabetes Federation estimates that countries are already spending between 6 and almost 17% of their annual healthcare expenditures on diabetes.[6]

The Lancet Commission on Global Mental Health and Sustainable Development estimates that the economic losses to the global economy from mental health disorders will be about $16 trillion from 2010 to 2030.[22]

Unfortunately, very little information is available about the economic costs of vision and hearing loss, especially in low- and middle-income countries. A report by the National Cancer Institute of the United States, in collaboration with WHO, concluded that the total economic costs of smoking to the world economy in 2012 were $1.4 trillion, or 1.8% of the world's GDP. The direct healthcare costs of smoking in 2012 were $422 billion, or approximately 5.7% of all healthcare expenditures that year.[37]

The limited studies that have been done on the costs of alcohol abuse can only be considered indicative because they did not follow any standard methodology. However, they all reveal substantial costs of alcohol abuse, as a share of GDP: Canada: 1.1%; France: 1.4%; Italy: 5.6%; and New Zealand: 4.0%.[38]

Addressing the Burden of Noncommunicable Diseases

The Global NCD Action Plan, endorsed by the World Health Assembly in 2013, lays out a series of evidence-based, cost-effective measures that are "best buys" in addressing the burden of some of the most important NCDs other than mental disorders. The most significant of these measures include excise taxes, laws on smoke-free zones, and the banning of advertising for tobacco products; a similar set of measures for alcohol; measures to reduce salt intake, eliminate trans fats, and promote better diets and physical activity; drug therapy to reduce the risks of CVD and diabetes; and hepatitis B immunization and prevention of cervical cancer to reduce the burden of cancers.[39] More recently, a WHO report of a high-level commission on NCDs recommended a number of best buys for the control of NCDs that focused on CVD, COPD, and diabetes.[40]

Additional Comments on Addressing Key Risk Factors for CVD, COPD, and Diabetes

Tobacco Use

The Framework Convention on Tobacco, agreed upon in 2003, outlines the measures that countries have agreed to undertake to reduce both the demand for and the supply of tobacco.[41] WHO then elaborated on these measures by outlining the MPOWER program for tobacco control, which consists of six elements: monitor tobacco use and prevention policies; protect people from tobacco smoke; offer help to quit tobacco use; warn about the dangers of tobacco use; enforce bans on tobacco advertising, promotion, and sponsorship; and raise taxes on tobacco.[40]

Alcohol

Despite the high burden of disease and economic costs that are related to excessive drinking of alcoholic beverages, very few countries have embarked on coherent efforts to reduce alcohol consumption. Those that have done so generally focused their attention on policy and legislative actions, such as taxation, laws on drunk driving, and restricting alcohol sales to selected places, times, and age limits. Controlled advertising and tightened law enforcement, such as through more widespread breath testing of drivers, have also been imposed. Another successful part of such programs was to encourage counseling by healthcare providers through "brief interventions with individual high-risk drinkers."[34]

High Blood Pressure, High Cholesterol, and Obesity

To reduce the burden of CVD and diabetes, healthy eating and maintaining a healthy weight are key. Generally, this requires eating more fruits and vegetables and decreasing the intake of salt and foods that are high in saturated fats and trans fats. It also entails limiting the intake of sugar and replacing refined grains with whole grains. People who are overweight generally need to consume fewer calories each day and need to become more active physically.[42] Tax policies can be used to subsidize healthier foods and tax those who are less healthy.

Countries can use public policies to try to limit the role of automobiles, promote walking and biking, and design communities in ways that encourage healthy lifestyles. In Singapore and London, for example, taxes are levied on cars that enter the center of the city to reduce the use of vehicles and their attendant traffic and pollution. Many cities, such as Amsterdam, promote the use of bicycles and have bicycle lanes.[42]

One way to promote healthier diets is through population-based health education. Large-scale education efforts of this type, often through mass media, have had mixed results because it is difficult to successfully promote the reduction of obesity on a large scale.[43] Generally, mass programs are more effective when they are combined with direct communication with individuals.

Even as countries undertake the steps noted, they will still need to treat those who already have CVD or who have some of the key risk factors for CVD, including hypertension. Most low-income countries and some middle-income countries do not have the level of health system or the financial resources needed to carry out sophisticated medical procedures. In such settings, however, an important reduction in risks and in the burden of disease can be realized through preventive interventions, such as getting people with high cholesterol and hypertension to take inexpensive medicines to lower blood pressure and cholesterol.[43]

Additional Comments on Addressing Diabetes, Cancer, Mental Health, and Vision and Hearing Loss

Further Addressing Diabetes

Avoiding overweight and obesity is the single most important way to prevent type 2 diabetes. Although large-scale efforts to reduce obesity have generally not been very successful, a pilot project that used intensive personal counseling to promote weight loss through healthier eating and more physical activity was successfully carried out in China, Finland, Sweden, and the United States. The average weight loss after almost 3 years of participation in this study was about 10 pounds more than in the control group. In addition, the study group had a 58% lower rate of type 2 diabetes than the control group.[12]

Treatment for people with diabetes is needed in all countries. For people with diabetes, it is cost-effective to control hypertension because the combination of the two diseases can produce major vascular complications. People with diabetes are also subject to foot problems from circulation difficulties associated with their diabetes, so appropriate foot care is another cost-effective investment.[12] Those countries with greater resources and a health system that can deliver additional interventions can also consider other cost-effective measures for treating diabetes, including vaccination against influenza and pneumococcal infections, diagnosis and treatment of retinal problems associated with diabetes, and treating hypertension with ACE inhibitors to prevent kidney problems from getting worse.[12]

Cancer

Tobacco control is overwhelmingly the first priority for preventing cancer, as noted earlier. Countries should also try to reduce the burden of cancer by vaccinating against infectious agents that are associated with cancers, such as hepatitis B and HPV, as an increasing number of countries are doing.[44]

The importance of prevention and early detection in low- and middle-income countries is highlighted by the fact that the stage of cancer at the time of detection in these countries is, on average, substantially more advanced than in wealthier countries. In some countries, in fact, as much as 80% of cancers may already be incurable when first diagnosed.[44] Although screening is possible for a number of cancers, DCP3 has suggested that only opportunistic screening for cervical cancer is generally cost-effective and manageable in low-income settings. However, that study also suggested that screening for some other cancers, such as oral cancers in places with a high prevalence rate of such cancers, might also be warranted.[44]

Even considering the present limitations on cancer treatment in a number of settings, DCP3 has suggested that it is cost-effective in low-resource settings to treat precancerous lesions of the cervix and to treat early-stage cervical, breast, and colorectal cancers. DCP3 also suggests that low-resource countries should seek to treat those childhood cancers that have high cure rates, a recommendation that goes beyond those of WHO.[44] Another aspect of cancer treatment is palliative care, which needs strengthening in most settings.[45]

Mental Health

There is generally an inadequate understanding of the importance of mental health, a lack of funds for mental health, a shortage of people who understand mental health issues, and stigma around mental disorders. In addition, the more limited the resources of a country, the wider the gaps are likely to be between what is needed to address mental disorders and what is available to do so.[20] Moreover, a significant amount of the mental health care in low- and middle-income countries is offered in large psychiatric hospitals that consume an overwhelming share of the mental health budget in those countries.

Yet, a range of mental disorders can be prevented and treated effectively outside of such settings. In fact, the evidence is growing that for $3 to $4 per person per year, countries could provide more community-based approaches to care that would offer drug therapy combined with psychosocial support for bipolar disorder, depression, and schizophrenia, as well as drug therapy for panic disorder.[46,]

Approaches that are cost-effective, scalable, and sustainable will have to depend on the community and on family-based efforts. In this light, and with increasing attention to mental disorders, in 2013 WHO published the *Mental Health Action Plan, 2013–2020.*[47] Some of the key recommended actions in the plan include the following: countries should have national plans for and laws on mental health that are consistent with international human rights; services for people with severe mental disorders should be increased by 20% and steps taken to reduce suicide by 10% by 2020; and countries should implement multisectoral mental health promotion and prevention programs and should improve their collection of and reporting on key mental health indicators. Unfortunately, no summary assessment of progress against this plan has been published.

The plan also recommended that countries should involve a broader range of stakeholders in their work on mental health, including those affected by mental disorders; shift services away from long-stay mental hospitals and toward community-based and evidenced-based approaches and community support; provide care that brings together promotion, prevention, care, and support; and reduce disparities by paying particular attention to groups most in need.[47]

Vision Loss

In 2013, the World Health Assembly approved a global action plan for universal eye health.[48]

The plan sets a target of reducing preventable blindness globally by 2019, from the 2010 baseline. The plan encourages countries to establish comprehensive eyecare programs that are well integrated into their health systems and that focus on cost-effective interventions to address refractive errors and the burden of unoperated cataracts. The plan also encourages countries to continue to work across sectors to help address the infectious and parasitic causes of blindness, as well as the growing threat of blindness related to diabetes. Eyecare is an area in which there has been considerable success with task shifting. This could include for eyecare, for example, ophthalmic assistants who are trained to do cataract surgeries, especially in places where there are an insufficient number of ophthalmologists. No summary of progress against this plan has been published. However, there was recently a Lancet Global Health Commission on Global Eye Care that follows up on the WHO report and lays out the next steps needed in global eye care.[49]

Hearing Loss

Despite the substantial burden of disease and economic costs related to hearing loss, the world has not yet adopted any coherent plan or targets to address this problem. WHO suggests, however, that about half of all cases of hearing loss can be addressed by primary prevention: immunizing children against measles, meningitis, rubella, and mumps; immunizing adolescent girls and women against rubella before pregnancy; improving antenatal and postnatal care, including screening for and treating syphilis and other infections in pregnant women; avoiding ototoxic drugs unless prescribed and monitored by a qualified physician; referring babies with high risk factors for early hearing assessment; and reducing both occupational and recreational exposure to loud noises through awareness, personal protective devices, and legislation.

WHO also suggests that attention be paid to early diagnosis and appropriate medical or surgical intervention for middle ear infections that can lead to hearing loss.[29] For that part of hearing loss that cannot be addressed through primary prevention, or for which it is too late, WHO recommends that countries focus on early detection of hearing loss, accompanied by appropriate management of the problem.[29]

Comments on the Usually Forgotten Oral Health

The Burden of Disease

Despite the enormous amount of disability related to oral disorders, such disorders have never been part of mainstream discussions of global health. In fact, seven oral diseases and conditions account for most of the oral disease burden globally: dental caries (tooth decay), periodontal (gum) diseases, oral cancers, oral manifestations of HIV, oro-dental trauma, cleft lip and palate, and Noma.[50] Yet, these diseases and conditions are either largely preventable or can be treated in their early stages.[50]

Oral diseases were estimated by GBD 2019 to have affected at least 3.48 billion people worldwide in 2019.[50] Caries of the permanent teeth were the most prevalent of all conditions assessed.[50] It was estimated that 2.4 billion people suffered from caries of permanent teeth and that almost 500 million children suffered from caries of primary teeth.[51]

In fact, "oral disorders," as they are called in GBD 2019, are among the most common of the noncommunicable diseases. Oral diseases were the tenth leading cause of years of life lived with disability (YLD) globally for all ages and both sexes in 2019. Oral disorders were the ninth leading cause of YLD globally for people 50 to 69 years of age and the tenth for people over 70 years of age.[2]

Dental caries and **periodontal disease** are two prominent but often neglected burdens of disease in low- and middle-income countries.[51] Dental caries, commonly known as tooth decay or cavities, are present in 90% of the global population, including an estimated 60 to 90% of all school-aged children worldwide.[51] Severe forms of periodontal disease affect 5 to 15% of most populations,[51] including approximately 2% of youth worldwide who suffer from juvenile or early-onset aggressive periodontitis.[51]

Dental caries and periodontal disease can lead to tooth loss. This is a very important cause of years of life lived with disability in countries with a large share of older people in their population. Moreover, both dental caries and periodontal disease contribute to childhood morbidity and have a negative impact on their quality of life.[52] Malnutrition prevalence rates also increase if children are too pained to eat.[53] A child's psychosocial well-being and ability to smile and speak may also be impaired.[47]

Another oral health disease of importance is Noma. This condition originates as an untreated gingival inflammation, which then evolves into a **gangrenous** lesion that causes necrosis of the lips, chin, and facial tissues.[54] The progression of Noma can be halted when it is detected at an early stage and treated appropriately. Such treatment would include good hygiene, antibiotics, and nutritional rehabilitation. Yet, it has been estimated that 90% of children who are exposed to this illness die as a result of receiving no medical care,[54] and survivors in those settings must often cope with severe facial disfigurement.[54]

Risk Factors for Dental Caries, Periodontal Disease, and Noma

There are a number of risk factors for dental caries, periodontal disease, and Noma in low- and middle-income countries. These include low education levels, low socioeconomic status, poor oral hygiene practices, alcohol and tobacco use, and excessive intake of dietary sugars. Diabetes is also thought to be linked with periodontitis in reciprocal ways.[51,54]

Barriers to Treatment and Prevention

In resource-poor countries, almost all tooth decay goes untreated.[55] The dental healthcare workforce in these countries is insufficient to satisfy service needs or demands.[52] Dentists in low-resource settings also tend to practice in urban settings. Another barrier to treatment is the high cost of dental services.[56]

There is strong evidence that long-term, low exposure to fluoride reduces the prevalence of dental caries in children.[52] However, successful implementation is largely contingent on the capacity of infrastructure of the affected population, and most low- and middle-income countries lack the resources to accomplish this.[52] Moreover, even on a household level in the lowest-income countries, fluoridated toothpaste can exceed a family's budget.[52]

Addressing Oral Health Issues

Interventions focused on cost-effective prevention methods that combine social policy and individual action will have the most impact in low- and middle-income countries.[57] It will be important to include oral health within the scope of comprehensive chronic disease prevention programs.[55] Government programs supporting subsidy and taxation relief of fluoridated toothpaste can also help address financial barriers.[52] Emphasis also needs to be placed on strengthening oral health education and promotional methods in community and school settings.[58]

Unintentional Injuries

Key Definitions

This section pays particular attention to the largest causes of **unintentional injury**, including road injuries. It does not cover all categories of injury included in the Global Burden of Disease Study, 2019.[2] It makes no comments about violence or self-harm, which was covered in the section on mental health.

The Importance of Injuries

Injuries are an important cause of deaths and DALYs in all regions of the world. In 2019, 7.6% of all deaths and 9.8% of all DALYs were attributable to injuries. In addition, these injuries are major causes of disability, with many people being disabled by injuries, even if they do not die from them. Moreover, the rate of deaths from injuries is substantially higher in low- and middle-income countries than in high-income countries.[2]

The Burden of Injuries

The leading cause of both deaths and DALYs attributable to injuries globally is road traffic injuries. Approximately 2.1% of all deaths and 2.9% of all DALYs globally are attributable to road injuries. This is followed by deaths from falls, drowning, poisoning, and fires.[2] The distribution of deaths from injuries varies by country income group. In high-income countries, deaths due to falls are greater than deaths from road injuries. However, in low-income countries, approximately five times as many deaths are attributable to road injuries as to falls.[2] About three times as many men die in road traffic accidents as women.[2] The number of deaths from road traffic accidents as a share of total deaths is particularly high in the Middle East and North Africa regions compared with other regions.[2]

Key Risk Factors

The key risk factors for injuries to children are developmental immaturity relative to the dangers children face, the influence of poverty on gaps in adult supervision, and exposure to unsafe workplaces.[59-62] The risk factors for road traffic injuries revolve around education, enforcement, and engineering. The risk factors of other leading causes of unintentional injuries relate largely to lower socioeconomic status, inadequate supervision of children, lack of safe storage of poisons, and household cooking arrangements that pay insufficient attention to fire hazards in areas that tend to be crowded and hazardous.[63]

The Costs and Consequences of Injuries

Although there have been few studies of the economic costs of injuries in low- and middle-income countries, estimates of such costs for road traffic injuries alone suggest that they range from 2 to 4% of GNP.[64-66] The social costs of dealing with the disabilities caused by accidents can also be very high. Numerous studies have documented the long-term physical and psychological consequences of unintentional injuries.[67,68]

Addressing Key Injury Issues

The importance of injuries to the overall burden of disease suggests that many countries need to put a greater priority on raising awareness of injuries and applying rigorous methods to the prevention and control of injuries.[69,70] There is increasing evidence from a range of countries of measures that can be taken to improve vehicle operator safety, build safety into vehicles, make plans for land use and traffic, and enforce key traffic rules.

These measures can be implemented in a phased manner in low- and middle-income countries and adapted to local settings. Reducing the burden of other injuries will also require enhancing community-based approaches to providing information about how the community can reduce risk factors for such injuries.[63] This could include, for example, education about storing poisons and giving families childproof storage containers.[71] To reduce injuries from falls will require attention to better supervision and play equipment for the young and working on balance and reducing home risk factors for the elderly. There is little information about cost-effective measures to reduce drowning among children beyond the need to enhance parental supervision. Strengthening emergency medical services can also be helpful to reducing the burden of deaths and disability from injuries.[72,73]

Discussion Questions

1. What is a noncommunicable disease? How does it differ from a communicable disease? What noncommunicable diseases have communicable causes?
2. What are the leading burdens of noncommunicable disease globally? How do these burdens vary across country income groups?
3. What are some of the most cost-effective and evidence-based measures to reduce the burden of cardiovascular disease and diabetes?
4. What measures might be taken in cost-effective ways to address mental disorders in low resource settings with few trained mental health professionals?
5. What are the leading burdens of unintentional injuries globally and what can be done in cost-effective ways in low-income countries to reduce those burdens?

References

1. The Lancet. *Global burden of disease*. 2019. Available at: https://www.thelancet.com/gbd#2019GBDIssue
2. Institute of Health Metrics and Evaluation (IHME). GBD Compare: Viz Hub. nd. Retrieved from https://vizhub.healthdata.org/gbd-compare/
3. Gaziano TA, Srinath Reddy K, Paccaud F, Horton S, Chaturvedi V. Cardiovascular disease. In: Jamison DT, Breman JG, Measham AR, et al., eds. *Disease control priorities in developing countries*. 2nd ed. Washington, DC: The World Bank; 2006:645–662.
4. World Heart Federation, World Stroke Federation. 2011. *Global atlas on cardiovascular disease prevention and control*. Retrieved from https://world-heart-federation.org/wp-content/uploads/2021/04/Global-Atlas-on-cardiovascular-disease-prevention-and-control.pdf
5. National Institutes of Health (NIH). *Obesity, physical activity, and weight control glossary*. nd. Retrieved from http:// win.niddk.nih.gov/publications/glossary.htm
6. International Diabetes Federation. (2017). *IDF diabetes atlas*. 8th ed. 2017. Retrieved from http://www.diabetesatlas.org/IDF_Diabetes_Atlas_8e_interactive_EN/
7. International Diabetes Federation. *IDF 2019 atlas*. 2019. Retrieved from https://www.diabetesatlas.org/en/

8. International Diabetes Federation. *Diabetes facts and figures.* 2020. Retrieved from https://www.idf.org/aboutdiabetes/what-is-diabetes/facts-figures.html

9. Ryerson B, Tierney EF, Thompson TJ, et al. Excess physical limitations among adults with diabetes in the U.S. population, 1997–1999. *Diabetes Care.* 2003;26(1):206–210.

10. International Diabetes Federation. *IDF diabetes atlas.* 6th ed. Brussels, Belgium: 2013.

11. Haffner SM. Epidemiology of type 2 diabetes: risk factors. *Diabet Care.* 1998;21(suppl 3):C3–C6.

12. Venkat Narayan K, Zhang P, Kanaya AM, et al. Diabetes: the pandemic and potential solutions. In: Jamison DT, Breman JG, Measham AR, et al., eds. *Disease control priorities in developing countries.* 2nd ed. Washington, DC: The World Bank; 2006:591–603.

13. World Health Organization (WHO). *Chronic obstructive pulmonary disease (COPD).* nd. Retrieved from https://www.who.int/respiratory/copd/en/

14. World Health Organization (WHO). *Chronic obstructive pulmonary Disease (COPD): Key facts.* 2017. Retrieved from https://www.who.int/en/news-room/fact-sheets/detail/chronic-obstructive-pulmonary-disease-(copd)

15. World Health Organization (WHO). *Cancer: key facts.* 2018A. Retrieved from https://www.who.int/en/news-room/fact-sheets/detail/cancer

16. International Agency for Research on Cancer. *Latest world global cancer statistics* (Press Release No. 233). Lyon, France; 2013.

17. Torre LA, Siegel RL, Ward EM, Jemal A. Global cancer incidence and mortality rates and trends—an update. *Cancer Epidemiol Biomarkers Prev.* 2016;25(1):16–27. doi:10.1158/1055-9965.EPI-15-0578

18. Veneis P, Wild CP. Global cancer patterns: causes and prevention. *The Lancet.* 2013;383(9916):549–557.

19. Centers for Disease Control and Prevention (CDC). *Parasites: schistosomiasis.* 2012. Retrieved from http://www.cdc.gov/parasites/schistosomiasis/index.html

20. World Health Organization (WHO). *Mental health: a state of well-being.* 2014. Retrieved from https://www.who.int/features/factfiles/mental_health/en/

21. Patel V, Chisholm D, Dua T, Laxminarayan R, Medina-Mora ME. Mental, neurological, and substance use disorders. In: Jamison DT, Gelband H, Horton S, et al., eds. *Disease Control Priorities.* 3rd ed. Washington, DC: World Bank; 2015: 4.

22. Patel V, Saxena S, Lund C, et al. *The Lancet* Commission on Global Mental Health and Sustainable Development. *Lancet Commissions,* 2018;392(10157):1553–1598.

23. WHO. *Blindness and vision impairment.* 2020. Retrieved from https://www.who.int/news-room/fact-sheets/detail/blindness-and-visual-impairment

24. World Health Organization (WHO). *Visual impairment and blindness* (Fact Sheet No. 282). 2014B. Retrieved from http://www.who.int/mediacentre/factsheets/fs282/en/

25. World Health Organization (WHO). *Blindness and vision impairment: key facts.* 2018B. Retrieved from https://www.who.int/en/news-room/fact-sheets/detail/blindness-and-visual-impairment

26. Cook J, Frick KD, Baltussen R, et al. Loss of vision and hearing. In: Jamison DT, Breman JG, Measham AR, et al., eds. *Disease control priorities in developing countries.* 2nd ed. Washington, DC: The World Bank; 2006: 953–962.

27. Flaxman SR, Bourne RRA, Resnikoff S, et al. Global causes of blindness and distance vision impairment 1990–2020: a systematic review and meta-analysis. *Lancet Glob Health.* 2017;5(12):e1221–1234.

28. World Health Organization (WHO). *Deafness and hearing loss: key facts.* 2018C. Retrieved from https://www.who.int/en/news-room/fact-sheets/detail/deafness-and-hearing-loss

29. World Health Organization (WHO). *WHO global estimates on prevalence of hearing loss.* 2012. Retrieved from https://www.who.int/pbd/deafness/WHO_GE_HL.pdf

30. Jha P, Chaloupka FJ, Moore J, et al. Tobacco addiction. In: Jamison DT, Breman JG, Measham AR, et al., eds. *Disease control priorities in developing countries.* 2nd ed. Washington, DC: The World Bank; 2006: 869–885.

31. Jha P, MacLennan M, Yurekli A, et al. Global hazards of tobacco and the benefits of smoking cessation and tobacco tax. In: Jamison DT, Gelband H, Horton S, et al., eds. *Disease Control Priorities.* 3rd ed. Washington, DC: The World Bank; 2015: 3.

32. World Health Organization (WHO). Tobacco: key facts. 2018. Retrieved from https://www.who.int/en/news-room/fact-sheets/detail/tobacco

33. Jamison DT, Breman JG, Measham AR, et al., eds. *Priorities in health.* Washington, DC: The World Bank; 2006.

34. Rehm J, Chisholm D, Room R, Lopez AD. Alcohol. In: Jamison DT, Breman JG, Measham AR, et al., eds. *Disease control priorities in developing countries.* 2nd ed. Washington, DC: The World Bank; 2006: 887–906.

35. Bloom DE, Cafiero ET, Jané-Llopis E, et al. *The global economic burden of noncommunicable diseases.* Geneva, Switzerland: World Economic Forum; 2011.

36. Jan S, Laba T-L, Essue, BM, et al. Action to address the household economic burden of non-communicable diseases. *Lancet.* 2018;391(10134):2047–2058.

37. World Health Organization (WHO). *Saving lives, spending less: a strategic response to noncommunicable diseases.* Geneva, Switzerland: 2018.

38. World Health Organization (WHO). *Global status report on alcohol 2004.* Geneva, Switzerland: 2004.

39. World Health Organization (WHO). *Global action plan for the prevention and control of noncommunicable diseases, 2013–2020.* Geneva, Switzerland; 2013A.

40. World Health Organization (WHO). *Time to deliver: report of the independent WHO high-level commission on noncommunicable diseases.* Geneva, Switzerland; 2018F.

41. Conference of the Parties to the WHO FCTC.IH, *WHO framework convention on tobacco control.* Geneva, Switzerland: World Health Organization; 2003.

42. Willett WC, Koplan JP, Nugent R, Dusenbury C, Puska P, Gaziano TA. Prevention of chronic disease by means of diet and lifestyle changes. 2006. In: Jamison DT, Breman JG, Measham AR, et al. (eds.), *Disease control priorities in developing countries* 2nd ed., pp. 833–850. Washington, DC: The World Bank.

43. Rodgers A, Lawes CM, Gaziano TA, Vos T. The growing burden of risk from high blood pressure, cholesterol, and bodyweight. In: Jamison DT, Breman JG, Measham AR, et al., eds. *Disease control priorities in developing countries.* 2nd ed. Washington, DC: The World Bank; 2006: 859–868.

44. Gelband H, Jha P, Sankaranarayanan R, Horton S. Cancer. In: Jamison DT, Gelband H, Horton S, et al., eds. *Disease Control Priorities.* 3rd ed. Washington, DC: The World Bank; 2015: 3.

45. Cleary J, Gelband H, Wagner J. *Cancer Pain Relief.* In: *Disease control priorities* (3rd edition): Volume 3, *Cancer,* Gelband H, Jha P, Sankaranarayanan R, Horton S, eds. Washington, DC: World Bank.

46. Patel V, Araya R, Chatterjee S, et al. Treatment and prevention of mental disorders in low-income and middle-income countries. *Lancet.* 2007;370(9591):991–1005.

47. World Health Organization (WHO). *Mental health action plan, 2013–2020.* Geneva, Switzerland: 2013.

48. World Health Organization (WHO). *Universal eye health: a global action plan 2014–2019.* Geneva, Switzerland: 2013.

49. Burton MJ, Ramke J, Marques AP, et al. The Lancet Global Health Commission on Global Eye Care. *Lancet Global Health.* 2021;9:e459–481.

50. Kassenbaum N, Hernandez C, Bailey J. Global, regional, and national levels and trends in burden of oral conditions from 1990 to 2017: a systematic analysis for the Global Burden of Disease 2017 study. *J Dent Res.* 2020. Retrieved May 4, 2021. http://www.healthdata.org/research-article/global-regional-and-national-levels-and-trends-burden-oral-conditions-1990-2017. doi:10.1177/0022034520908533

51. World Health Organization (WHO). *Oral health: key facts.* 2018. Retrieved from https://www.who.int/news-room/fact-sheets/detail/oral-health

52. The Lancet. Oral health: prevention is key. *Lancet.* 2009;373(9657), 1. doi: 10.1016/S0140-6736(08)61933-9

53. World Health Organization (WHO). (2014). *What is the burden of oral disease?* Retrieved from http://www.who.int

54. Enwonwu CO, Falkler WA, Phillips RS. Noma (cancrum oris). *Lancet,* 2006;368(9530): 147–156. doi: 10.1016/S0140-6736(06)69004-1

55. Benzian H, Hobdell M, Mackay J. Putting teeth into chronic diseases. *Lancet.* 2011; 377(9764):464. doi: 10.1016/S0140-6736(11)60154-2

56. World Health Organization (WHO). (2014). *What is the burden of oral disease?* Retrieved from http://www.who.int

57. Evert J, Drain PK, Hall T. Vignette: Dr. Karen Sokal-Gutierrez and the Children's Oral Health Nutrition Project. In: *Developing global health programming: a guidebook for medical and professional schools.* San Francisco, CA: Global Health Education Collaborations Press; 2014: 219–220.

58. Children's Dental Health Project. (2013). *Cost effectiveness of preventive dental services.* Retrieved from https://www.cdhp.org/resources/163-cost-effectiveness-of-preventive-dental-services

59. Jordan J, Valdez-Lazo F. Education on safety and risk. In: Manciaux M, Romer C, eds. *Accidents in childhood and adolescence: the role of research.* Geneva, Switzerland: World Health Organization; 1991: 106–120.

60. Ljungblom B-A, Köhler L. Child development and behavior in traffic. In: Manciaux M, Romer C, eds. *Accidents in childhood and adolescence: the role of research.* Geneva, Switzerland: World Health Organization; 1991: 97–105.

61. Leflamme L, Diderichsen F. Social differences in traffic injury risk in childhood and youth—a literature review and a research agenda. *Injury Prevention.* 2000;6: 293–298.

62. International Labour Office. *Child labour: targeting the intolerable.* Geneva, Switzerland: International Labour Office; 1996.

63. Norton R, Hyder AA, Bishai D, Peden, M. Unintentional injuries. In: Jamison DT, Breman JG, Measham AR, et al., eds. *Disease control priorities in developing countries.* 2nd ed. New York, NY: Oxford University Press; 2006: 737–753.

64. Rezaei S, Arab M, Matin BK, Sari AA. Extent, consequences and economic burden of road crashes in Iran. *Journal of Injury and Violence Research* 2014;6(2):57–63.

65. Ghadi M, Török Á., Tánczos K. Study of the economic cost of road accidents in Jordan. *Periodica Polytechnica Transportation Engineering.* 2018;46(3):129–134.

66. Mohan D. *Impact of road traffic crashes in Asia: a human and economic assessment.* United Nations Centre for Regional Development. 2014. Retrieved from https://www.researchgate.net /publication/274075965_IMPACT_OF_ROAD_TRAFFIC_CRASHES_IN_ASIA_A_HUMAN _AND_ECONOMIC_ASSESSMENT

67. Mayou R, Bryant B. Outcome in consecutive emergency department attenders following a road traffic accident. *British Journal of Psychiatry.* 2001;179(6):528–534.

68. Osberg J, Khan P, Rowe K, Brooke MM. Pediatric trauma: impact on work and family finances. *Pediatrics.* 1996;98(5):890–897.

69. Bartlett SN. The problem of children's injuries in low-income countries: a review. *Health Pol Plan.* 2002;17(1):1–13.

70. Haddon, W. (1999). The changing approach to epidemiology, prevention, and amelioration of trauma: the transition to approaches etiologically rather than descriptively based. *Injury Prevention.* 1999;5:231–235.

71. Krug A, Ellis JB, Hay IT, Mokgabudi NF, Robertson J. The impact of child-resistant containers on the incidence of paraffin (kerosene) ingestion in children. *South African Medical Journal.* 1994;84(11):730–734.

72. Mock C, Arreola-Risa, C, Quansah R. Strengthening care for injured persons in less developed countries: a case study of Ghana and Mexico. *Injury Control and Safety Promotion.* 2003; 10(1-2):45–51.

73. Kobusingye OC, Hyder AA, Bishai D, Joshipura ERH, Mock C. Emergency medical services. In: Jamison DT, Breman JG, Measham AR, et al., eds. *Disease control priorities in developing countries.* 2nd ed. New York, NY: Oxford University Press; 2006: 1261–1279.

Epilogue

The book ends as it began, by highlighting why the study of global health is so important. The Introduction suggested that:

- The health of anyone, anywhere, is the health of everyone, everywhere. Diseases don't respect boundaries.
- There is an ethical dimension to questions concerning the extent to which all people can lead a healthy and productive life, in fair ways.
- Health is closely linked with social and economic productivity.
- Health and well-being have important links with security and freedom.
- Some global health issues require global cooperation, such as the need for pandemic preparedness and response, vaccine development, and vaccine deployment across countries.

The coronavirus pandemic that began in 2019 reminds us in stark ways of the importance of each of these points:

- The outbreak appears to have begun in China at the end of 2019 but spread quickly throughout the world. By early July 2021, almost 185 million people worldwide had tested positive for the virus and more than 4 million people had died from it.[1]
- The pandemic highlighted an array of ethical issues related to mask wearing, store closings, and the impact of the pandemic on minority communities. It also highlighted ethical issues related to the distribution of scarce vaccines. How should the limited vaccine doses that are available be distributed within and across countries? What principles should guide distribution? Is it fair for high-income countries to have bought up so much of the available supply, leaving other countries waiting to vaccinate their people?
- The economic and social costs of the pandemic have been beyond measure. The pandemic led to the shutting down of a wide variety of economic activities in many countries. It led to school closings. Many people deferred medical care and got sick or died as a result. An early estimate suggested that the pandemic had already cost the United States $16 trillion.[2]
- The coronavirus also revealed major social and political cleavages in a number of countries. Some people supported public health measures they were asked to take. Others demonstrated against them. Some people supported the deployment of a vaccine. Others suggested that the vaccine was part of a plot by some people to harm other people.
- The pandemic made exquisitely clear the need for global cooperation. The world required from China timely and honest information at the start of the outbreak, which appears not to have been the case. On the other hand, the Chinese released the genome of the virus in a timely manner, which was

critical to efforts to develop tests and vaccines as early as possible. A test was developed, which WHO made available to any country that wanted it. Lessons were shared across countries on the clinical management of COVID-19 disease. Actors from many countries, in the public and private sectors, worked together to develop vaccines. Some countries also assisted others in creating a platform for sharing vaccines and for financing them. Effective action in each of these areas is central to the ability to control this pandemic. This will also be central to controlling future disease outbreaks.

In addition to preparing for other pandemics and the continuing threats of antimicrobial resistance, there remains a large unfinished agenda of actions needed to address nutrition, maternal and child health, and communicable diseases. There are also major gaps in dealing with noncommunicable diseases, mental health disorders, and injuries. In addition, climate change is a growing threat to global health.

Hopefully, this book has helped you gain a better understanding of whom critical global health issues affect; why they occur; why they are so important; and what we have learned can be done to address them in cost-effective, doable, sustainable, and fair ways.

There is much more to explore in the global health field. Interested readers could usefully begin such an exploration with readings on the history and governance of global health. Readers not already working in global health are also encouraged to learn more about professions in this exciting and exceptionally important arena.

References

1. Worldometer. *Covid-19 Coronavirus Pandemic.* (July 6, 2021). Retrieved from https://www.worldometers.info/coronavirus/.
2. Cutler DM, Summers LH. The COVID-19 pandemic and the $16 trillion virus. *JAMA.* 2020;324(15):1495–1496. doi:10.1001/jama.2020.19759

Glossary

A

Age dependency ratio The ratio between the number of people who are 15 to 64 years of age, compared with the number who are 65 years of age or older.

Ambient air Atmospheric air in its natural state.

Anxiety disorder A mental disorder in which feelings of worry or nervousness interfere with daily life.

B

Behavioral approach A component of combination prevention for HIV involving efforts to change people's behavior so they have less risk of becoming infected with HIV.

Behavioral change In health, this refers to changing people's behaviors so they engage in more health-enabling behaviors, such as giving up tobacco consumption or wearing seat belts.

Bipolar affective disorder A mood disorder that brings unusual shifts in mood, energy, activity levels, and the ability to carry out day-to-day tasks.

Biomedical approach A component of combination prevention for HIV infection involving interventions such as male medical circumcision, treating sexually transmitted infections, and antiretroviral therapy.

Burden of disease A term used to describe the combination of morbidity, disability, and mortality, usually measured in DALYs in global health work.

C

Case management (treatment) and improved caregiving An approach to communicable disease control (and for other health conditions) involving a collaborative process of assessment, planning, facilitation, care coordination, evaluation, and advocacy for options and services to meet an individual's and family's comprehensive health needs.

Case surveillance, reporting, and containment An approach to communicable disease control involving identification of cases, epidemiologic analysis, and systematic planning to immediately contain each case to eliminate the possibility of further transmission.

Child mortality rate The number of deaths of children under age five per 1,000 live births.

Chronic obstructive pulmonary disease (COPD) Chronic lung disease that causes limitations in lung airflow.

Climate change The increase in the earth's average temperature that has been observed and the consequences that might be associated with this rise in temperature.

Communicable diseases (also called infectious diseases) Illnesses that are caused by a particular infectious agent and that spread directly or indirectly from people to people, from animals to animals, from animals to people, or from people to animals.

D

Death rate (also called mortality rate) The number of deaths per 1,000 population in a given year.

Demographic Regarding the population's makeup.

Demographic transition The shift from high fertility and high mortality to low fertility and low mortality.

Dental caries Tooth decay or cavities.

Depression Clinical depression is a mood disorder in which feelings of sadness, loss, anger, or frustration interfere with activities of everyday life for a significant period of time.

Determinants of health The range of personal, social, economic, and environmental factors that determine the health status of individuals or populations.

Diabetes Medical illness caused by too little insulin or poor response to insulin.

Disability The temporary or long-term reduction in a person's capacity to function.

Disability-adjusted life year (DALY) A composite measure of premature deaths and losses due to disabilities in a population.

Drug resistance The extent to which infectious and parasitic agents develop an ability to resist drug treatment.

E

Emerging infectious disease A newly discovered infectious disease.

Environment External physical, chemical, and microbiological exposures and processes that impinge upon individuals and groups and are beyond the immediate control of individuals.

Environmental health A set of public health efforts that is implemented to prevent disease, death, and disability by reducing exposure to adverse environmental conditions and promoting behavior change. It focuses on the direct and indirect causes of disease and injuries and taps resources inside and outside of the healthcare system to help improve health outcomes.

Epidemiologic transition A shift in the pattern of disease from largely communicable diseases to noncommunicable diseases.

F

Female genital mutilation (also called female circumcision and female genital cutting) A collective term for various traditional practices that are all related to the cutting of the female genital organs; four different forms and grades are usually distinguished.

Foodborne (illness) A disease originating from the contamination of food.

Food security A state when people have availability and adequate access at all times to sufficient, safe, nutritious food to maintain a healthy and active life.

G

Gangranous Referring to a part of a person's body that is decaying because of a lack of blood flow.

Gestational diabetes or gestational diabetes mellitus (GDM) Diabetes that develops during pregnancy because of improper regulation of blood sugar; it usually goes away after delivery but can increase the woman's risk of developing type II diabetes later.

H

Health disparities Differences in health that are closely linked to social or economic disadvantage.

Health equity The absence of unfair and avoidable or remediable differences in health among different population groups.

Health impact assessment A combination of procedures, methods, and tools by which a policy, program, or project may be judged as to its potential effects on the health of a population and the distribution of those effects within the population.

Health inequity Differences in health that are not only unnecessary and avoidable but also unfair and unjust.

Health system The combination of resources, organization, and management that culminates in the delivery of health services to the population.

High-risk drinking Drinking 20 grams or more per day of pure alcohol for a woman and 40 grams a day for a man.

Hyperglycemia in pregnancy See gestational diabetes.

I

Improved care seeking, disease recognition An approach to controlling the spread of communicable disease involving enhancing people's ability to seek health care when they become infected, as well as improving people's ability to correctly recognize particular diseases.

Improved water, sanitation, hygiene A strategy for controlling the spread of communicable disease which involves providing safe access to clean water and sanitation, as well as promoting hygienic practices, such as handwashing.

Incidence rate The rate at which new cases of a disease occur in a population.

Induced abortion Premature expulsion or loss of embryo that is not spontaneous.

Inequality in health Differences in health status or in the distribution of health determinants between different population groups.

Infant mortality rate The number of deaths of infants under age 1 per 1,000 live births in a given year.

Inhalation A path of transmission of infectious disease involving the respiration of aerosolized droplets containing the infectious agent (e.g., tuberculosis, influenza, and meningitis).

Injuries The result of an act that damages, harms, or hurts; unintentional or intentional damage to the body resulting from acute exposure to thermal, mechanical, electrical, or chemical energy, or from the absence of such essentials as heat or oxygen.

Iron deficiency anemia Low level of hemoglobin in the blood.

Ischemic heart disease Also known as coronary heart disease and characterized by a reduced blood supply to the heart.

L

Life expectancy at birth The average number of years a newborn baby could expect to live if current mortality trends were to continue for the rest of the newborn's life.

Life table A representation of the probable years of survivorship of any population. For the Global Burden of Disease Study, there is a standard reference life table that takes account of the highest life expectancies at birth globally for males and for females and are used in calculations of years of life lost due to premature deaths.

Low birthweight Birthweight less than 2,500 grams.

M

Malnutrition Various forms of poor nutrition, including underweight, stunting, wasting, and overweight or obesity, as well as micronutrient deficiencies.

Mass chemotherapy A preventive form of mass administration of drug therapy to control infection.

Maternal mortality ratio The number of women who die as a result of pregnancy and childbirth complications per 100,000 live births in a given year.

Mental health A state of well-being in which every individual realizes her or his own potential, can cope with the normal stresses of life, can work productively and fruitfully, and is able to make a contribution to her or his community.

Micronutrient deficiencies A lack of the essential micronutrients required for good health.

Modifiable Lifestyle factors that can be changed.

Morbidity Illness.

Mortality Death.

N

Neonatal mortality rate Number of deaths of children under 28 days of age in a given year per 1,000 live births in that year.

Neonatal period The period from birth to 28 days of age.

Noncommunicable diseases Illnesses that are not spread by any infectious agent.

Nongovernmental organization A nonprofit group or association organized outside of institutionalized political structures to realize particular social objectives, such as environmental protection, or to serve particular constituencies, such as indigenous peoples.

Nontraumatic contact Contact with a certain infectious agent that can cause disease but does not require physical injury for entry (e.g., anthrax).

O

Obesity (for an adult) Body mass index over 30. For a child, the body mass index is greater or equal to the 95th percentile for minors of the same age and sex.

Obstetric fistula An injury in the birth canal that allows leakage from the bladder or rectum into the vagina, leaving a woman permanently incontinent, often leading to isolation and exclusion from the family and community.

Obstructed labor When the fetus cannot descend through the birth canal because of a blockage.

Occupational health A discipline that focuses on avoiding and reducing serious injuries and diseases among workers.

Occupational safety and health (OSH) The science of the anticipation, recognition, evaluation, and control of hazards arising in or from the workplace that could impair the health and well-being of workers.

One Health The integrative effort of multiple disciplines working locally, nationally, and globally to attain optimal health for people, animals, and the environment.

Overweight (for an adult) A body mass index between 25 and 30.

P

Pandemic preparedness The ability to effectively deal with a global outbreak of disease.

Periodontal disease An inflammatory disease that can affect the gums and bones that support the teeth and can lead to tooth loss.

Postneonatal period The period between 29 days and one year of age.

Prevalence The number of people suffering from a certain condition over a specific time period.

Primary care The provision of first contact, person-focused, ongoing care over time that meets the health-related needs of people.

R

Reemerging infectious disease An existing disease that has increased in incidence or has taken on new forms.

Replacement fertility The total fertility rate needed for a population to exactly replace itself from one generation to the next without migration.

Risk factor An aspect of personal behavior or lifestyle, an environmental exposure, or an inborn or inherited characteristic that, on the basis of epidemiologic evidence, is known to be associated with health-related conditions.

S

Safe abortion An abortion performed by personnel with the needed skills in accordance with methods recommended by WHO and in a manner appropriate for the length of the pregnancy.

Schizophrenia A chronic, severe, and disabling brain disorder.

Secondary care Medical care provided by a specialist or facility upon referral by a primary care physician.

Severely wasted An extreme form of malnutrition defined by a very low weight-for-height measurement of three z scores below the median WHO growth standards.

Sexual or bloodborne A path of transmission for certain communicable diseases (e.g., HIV, hepatitis) involving contact between blood, semen, vaginal fluid, or anal mucosa.

Social determinants of health The conditions in which people are born, grow, live, work, and age.

Stillbirth A baby who dies during or before birth but after 28 weeks of pregnancy.

Stroke Temporary or permanent loss of the blood supply to the brain.

Structural approach A component of combination prevention for HIV that addresses the underlying societal elements that predispose a person to the risk of infection.

Stunting Failure to reach linear growth potential because of inadequate nutrition or poor health; two z-scores below the international reference.

T

Task shifting The rational redistribution of tasks among health workforce teams. Specific tasks are moved, where appropriate, from highly qualified health workers to health workers with shorter training and fewer qualifications in order to make more efficient use of the available human resources for health.

Tertiary care Specialized consultative care, usually on referral from primary or secondary medical care personnel, by specialists working in a center that has personnel and facilities for special investigation and treatment.

Traumatic contact A scratch or bite through which certain infectious diseases can be spread (e.g., rabies).

U

Undernutrition A state of being underweight for one's age, too short for one's age (stunted), dangerously thin for one's height (wasted), or deficient in vitamins and minerals (micronutrient malnutrition).

Underweight Low weight-for-age; two z-scores below the international reference for weight-for-age.

Unintentional injury That subset of injuries for which there is no evidence of predetermined intent.

Universal health coverage Ensuring that all people can use the promotive, preventive, curative, rehabilitative, and palliative health services they need, of sufficient quality to be effective, while also ensuring that the use of these services does not expose the user to financial hardship.

V

Vaccination A biological preparation that improves immunity to a particular disease and typically contains an agent that resembles a disease-causing microorganism.

Vector-borne (diseases) Diseases transmitted through mosquitoes, sandflies, triatomine bugs, blackflies, ticks, tsetse flies, mites, snails, and lice.

Vector control A method to contain or totally eradicate any insects, rats, mammals, or disease-transmitting animals. Most commonly seen with mosquito control.

Viral load The number of viral particles found in each milliliter of blood.

W

WASH Water, sanitation, and hygiene.

Wasting Weight, measured in kilograms, divided by height in meters squared that is two z-scores below the international reference.

Waterborne (illness) A disease caused by drinking contaminated water.

Z

Zoonoses A disease that can be transmitted to humans from animals.

Index

Note: Page numbers followed by *f* or *t* represent figures or tables respectively.

F

G

H

I